Praise for *Mama, Mama, Only Mama*

"Lara Lillibridge's memoir, *Mama, Mama, Only Mama*, is a raw, honest, and very relatable tale of motherhood. I laughed, I cried, I shook my fist in solidarity. All moms out there need to read this one, even if your kids are grown or still in egg form. You won't regret it!"
—Whitney Dineen, author of *Motherhood, Martyrdom & Costco Runs*

"*Mama, Mama, Only Mama* is engaging, relatable, and addictive. All sorts of parents will love this unforgettable memoir. Since I'm the sort that enjoys belly laughs, it's the perfect fit."
—Terri Libenson, syndicated cartoonist of *The Pajama Diaries* and bestselling author of *Invisible Emmie* and *Positively Izzy*

"*Mama, Mama, Only Mama* is hilarious, achingly real, and one of those books that will end up being passed around the carpool line. You'll crack up, you'll relate, you'll wish you could hang out at Lara Lillibridge's house on Saturday afternoons."
—Lisa Daily, bestselling author of *Single-Minded*

"A delicious, open-hearted, delightful collection."
—Erin Judge, stand-up comedian and author of *Vow of Celibacy*

"An absolute must for single parents, at any stage. Lara Lillibridge's memoir, *Mama, Mama, Only Mama*, is hilarious, sweet, and hopeful. As a single mum myself, I could relate to almost every word—each page gave me strength, made me laugh and cry, and reminded me of what is important."
—Shannon Leone Fowler, author of *Traveling with Ghosts*

"Real, raw and ridiculously funny—Lara is the unabashedly honest mum we've all been waiting for."
—Amy Baker, author of *Miss-Adventures: A Tale of Ignoring Life Advice While Backpacking Around South America*

MAMA, MAMA, ONLY MAMA

MAMA, MAMA, ONLY MAMA

An Irreverent Guide for the Newly Single Parent—
From Divorce and Dating to Cooking and Crafting,
All While Raising the Kids and
Maintaining Your Own Sanity (Sort of)

Lara Lillibridge

Skyhorse Publishing

Skyhorse Publishing books may be purchased in bulk at special discounts for sales promotion, corporate gifts, fund-raising, or educational purposes. Special editions can also be created to specifications. For details, contact the Special Sales Department, Skyhorse Publishing, 307 West 36th Street, 11th Floor, New York, NY 10018 or info@skyhorsepublishing.com.

Skyhorse® and Skyhorse Publishing® are registered trademarks of Skyhorse Publishing, Inc.®, a Delaware corporation.

Visit our website at www.skyhorsepublishing.com.

10 9 8 7 6 5 4 3 2 1

Library of Congress Cataloging-in-Publication Data

Names: Lillibridge, Lara, author.
Title: Mama, mama, only mama: an irreverent guide for the newly single parent—from divorce and dating to cooking and crafting, all while raising the kids and maintaining your own sanity (sort of) / Lara Lillibridge.
Description: New York, New York: Skyhorse Publishing, Inc., [2019]
Identifiers: LCCN 2018033664 (print) | LCCN 2018037244 (ebook) | ISBN 9781510743571 (eBook) | ISBN 9781510743564 (hardcover: alk. paper)
Subjects: LCSH: Lillibridge, Lara. | Single mothers. | Parenting. | Children of divorced parents.
Classification: LCC HQ759.915 (ebook) | LCC HQ759.915 .L55 2019 (print) | DDC 306.874/32—dc23
LC record available at https://lccn.loc.gov/2018033664

Cover design by Mona Lin
Cover photo by iStockphoto

Print ISBN: 978-1-5107-4356-4
eBook ISBN: 978-1-5107-4357-1

Printed in China

For L. and R.,
the real-life Big and Tiny Pants
(No, you're not old enough to read it yet.)

Disclaimer: I'm not a chef. I'm not entirely sure what I do counts as cooking. What my family likes is not necessarily what your family likes, and as you will read, my family doesn't even like all the recipes contained herein. Proceed at your own risk: push up your sleeves, use oven mitts accordingly, and it never hurts to keep a fire extinguisher handy.

Excruciatingly Long Table of Contents
(I'm not kidding)

PART ONE
THE DISSOLUTION OF OUR MARRIAGE

Step Stools

Everyone wants to know why my marriage ended. It's a natural curiosity, I suppose, but it's not a question I want to answer. There's the easy answer, and the hard answer. Easy answers are all about what he or I did or didn't do, but they always end with, "yeah, but couldn't you have tried harder?"

Then there's the hard answer, which takes time to understand in my own head and longer still to codify for everyone else. Still, I should have an answer. Whether others find it satisfying or not is irrelevant.

To say why my marriage failed, I have to first talk about a pair of step stools of the same approximate size and shape. One is pale green, the color of a tulip stem. Made of lightweight, molded plastic, its design is clean, simple, functional. As far as step stools go, it is perfectly adequate. The other step stool is old wood, long ago painted red but now covered with paint splatter from other people's projects and also a few of my own. I cannot tell you why I had to buy it at that garage sale last summer, the one we walked to around the corner, where my youngest child bought a mini tape recorder and I found so many things that pleased me that I left with my arms overflowing. The red step stool was only one dollar, but I would have paid five or even ten dollars for it, even though I already had a perfectly adequate step stool at home. I couldn't live with new molded plastic once I found old wood painted red and worn in spots by years of other children's feet.

My ex-husband is a good man, but he will always choose the pale green step stool the color of tulip stems and our cat's eyes. When he looks at the old red wood stool, he sees only junk past its prime and destined for the garbage heap. When I look at the green plastic one, I see only cheap, prefabricated function-over-form nonsense. I told him when we met that I liked the plastic one better, that I wanted new and clean and functional, and I wanted to want that, I really did. But I woke up one day and saw that there was no old paint-splattered wood anywhere and I couldn't live like that anymore. There was no room for worn-down red in our fresh, new, and functional tract home filled with soft beige and ivory and a dash of pale blue.

My ex-husband will tell you that one day I woke up and had gone crazy, and nothing worked right after that no matter how hard he tried. His version is also true. What can you say to someone who sees old paint-splattered wood as junk without sounding crazy? How can you live without old wood and not become crazy?

When I go to my ex-husband's house now—the one we bought and furnished together—little has changed in the five years since I left. I left no lasting impression; I painted no walls, hung no art. That's not true. I sewed the throw pillows on the couch. I hung the posters in the playroom, the ones his sister sent. But what I did was so anonymous and bland it could have been done by anyone. I can't believe I ever lived like that. When my ex comes to my house—the one I have lived in for the last five years—it is overflowing with chaos and toy splatter and half-finished projects. He can't imagine anyone would want to live like this.

Swedish Meatballs

My mother and her wusband (woman-husband) are feminists. They view anything domestic as oppressive labor, including cooking.

When I was in high school I worked at a flower shop with a bunch of gay men. I was invited to my first gay (as opposed to lesbian) party. They had caviar. They had flower arrangements. They had sparkling glass bowls and tea light candles and all their food was displayed on little risers so everything was at a different height. I went home and called my mother in indignation.

"You aren't really gay!" I exclaimed.

"What do you mean I'm not gay?" she asked, somewhat justifiably flabbergasted.

"I went to a party at William's house and there was caviar and candles, and flowers, and all the food was up in risers on different heights. Your party food was cocktail weenies and Doritos in a basket lined with a paper towel!" My mother's laughter interrupted my rant.

"Oh, honey, you just learned the difference between gays and lesbians. Gay parties are Hollywood. Lesbian parties are Doritos in a basket."

I swore I wouldn't learn to cook from my mother. Instead, I learned the fine art of making Hamburger Helper from my high school boyfriend and pretty much everything else from my first husband: omelets, soup, pasta sauce from scratch. I was competent in the kitchen, but took no joy in it.

After my first divorce, I met my future second-ex-husband, whom my parents adored. This was the kind of man they had always dreamed of me marrying. He even had red hair—my stepmother's absolute favorite color that hair comes in. For my birthday, my parents gave me one of Betty Crocker's easy cookbooks so I could woo him properly. I was not thrilled. I knew how to cook, for fuck's sake. And the irony of my lesbian stepmother giving me man-trapping secrets was a record screech of a role-reversal.

"I'll teach you my secret recipe for Swedish meatballs," my stepmother told me with an evil/unstable/completely irrational gleam in her eye, "so you can cook it for your future-second-ex-husband!" Let the record reflect she had not ever made Swedish meatballs in my lifetime.

"Let me guess, you make meatballs and cook them in Campbell's Cream of Mushroom soup?" I answered, having never cooked them myself, but having a basic understanding of such things.

"And I add sour cream!" she purred.

"Let me get this right—my lesbian stepmother is giving me man-trapping secrets?" I asked.

"You should make sure your apartment is clean anytime he comes over," she answered.

I never made Swedish meatballs for my future-ex-second-husband, because he doesn't like Swedish meatballs. However, as a single mother, I made them all the freaking time, because it turns out that I do like Swedish meatballs, and they are wicked easy to make.

How to Make Swedish Meatballs

1. Buy Lean Cuisine Swedish Meatballs. All other brands are too salty.
2. Remove convenient plastic tray from box in such a way that you can save the box. This is important.
3. Stab package several times with sharp knife (or the scissors on your desk if you are at work) to vent the package and relieve some of your latent rage. If you do not have any latent rage you probably won't relate to anything in this book and might as well stop reading now. WARNING: control your rage to the degree that you do not pierce the convenient plastic serving tray.
4. Set the nicely stabbed/vented (but not too much) convenient plastic tray on top of the empty box inside the microwave. This facilitates airflow or maybe just adds magic.
5. Ignore the directions about 50 percent power blah blah blah. Just nuke the fucker on high for 4 minutes.
6. Remove from microwave, slide back into the box, and carry to your desk/table/sofa. This prevents you from burning your hands or spilling the contents on your shirt.
7. Remove plastic film and stuff inside box. Set convenient plastic tray on top of slightly flattened box which now doubles as a cheap placemat. Enjoy!

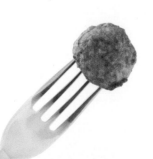

The Beginning Always Starts with an Ending

Mike "Daddy Pants" and I sat side by side on the smooth wooden bench. I remember it being blond wood—maple maybe—and slightly curved in the back. Hard, yes, but designed to be sat on for hours if needed. Luckily, we didn't need to wait that long. We whispered back and forth, making jokes about the lawyers and other people whose turn came before ours. I gave him a piece of gum. I wanted to reach out and touch his hand or playfully swat his thigh, but I couldn't, of course. We were waiting for our divorce hearing, and the casual intimacy of the moment was an unexpected respite from the previous months of arguing.

I'd say neither of us expected it would come to this, but no one ever goes into a marriage expecting to wind up in divorce court four years and two children later.

• • •

We'd started in the usual way—facing each other in front of a rented floral arch, bathed in Chicago's May light. I wanted to reach out and touch his hand that day, too, but everyone was watching, and I was suddenly shy. He glowed, but then, he had always glowed to me. His face was naturally ruddy, and sunlight found the tips of his crew-cut strawberry-blond hair and surrounded his face in halo, like a church painting. It was my sign that he was the right one for me. He was my beloved friend, the person I had chosen to stand beside in front of minister and family, gazing toward a future composed of children and white picket fences. I did not love him passionately, the way a wife should love her husband, but I told myself it didn't matter.

It was my second time down the aisle. My first marriage began when I was twenty years old, wearing a dress bought from the classifieds, and ended when I was twenty-six, driving with my stepmother from New York to Key West without much more than the clothes on my back, a Rottweiler in the back seat, and a cat that wouldn't stop howling.

• • •

Unlike my first husband, Mike was a man who didn't get into fistfights with strangers or make me cry until my head ached. He tolerated my family and made tinfoil hats for my cat to wear. Marriage seemed like the right thing to do—crazy love had almost destroyed me the first time around. I could not trust myself to free-fall into passion again. And he deserved someone who was overwhelmingly in love with him, and though I knew it was not me, still I said I would be his wife.

Whitefish Girl

My teenage years had earned me a reputation of being *easy*. *Easy* as in *yielding, promiscuous, achievable, unchaste*, yes, but also *easy* as in *straightforward, uninhibited, vulnerable*. My feminist upbringing left me naive—I did not know the rules of teenaged sexuality that everyone else seemed to follow. I didn't understand that my eyes were hungry, or that I stood too close to men when I talked to them. I was taught to never wait by the phone for a boy to call me, but instead to pursue whomever interested me. This turned me into a *boy-chaser*, a girl you didn't take home to your mother. I was incapable of being coy, and I was guileless, naive. Moreover, I wasn't raised to view sexual acts with shame, and this lack of shame translated into a lack of quality in other people's eyes.

I still don't understand how sexual eagerness translates into disgrace for a girl but prowess for a boy of the same age, and I'm not sure that I even want to anymore. I don't wish that I was cunning, evasive, or any of the other things that good girls need to be to remain un-dirty. I didn't want to say *no* when I meant *yes*. I didn't want to pretend to be browbeaten into having sex when it was something I wanted to do, just because some code insisted that's how good girls stayed clean.

Maybe the slut rules—which I was surprised to learn do not end in adolescence—are what we as a society should be ashamed of. Rules that say that a woman must be persuaded and pressured if she expects to both be sexually active and retain value. I wish that I had flouted the rules intentionally and with derision, instead of blindly. I wish that I had looked at those boys—the ones who touched me in the dark and called me slut in the light—and told them that they were not good enough to ever again touch my littlest toenail. Instead I said nothing and tried my best not to cry.

• • •

One year, a few friends of Mike's visited us in Key West. One man, who was married, had sex in a hot tub with a girl he had met at a bar that night. The other guys laughed when he told us, and called her "Coney Island Whitefish," whatever that meant. To have slept with someone who wanted to sleep with him, to have expected that a man without a ring on his finger was not married made her trash in their eyes. Was it because she slept with him on the first date, or because her face was acne-scarred? I listened to them mock and tease her after she left and I said nothing. The married man had kept her panties as a trophy, and he laughed when his friends threw them off our fourth-floor balcony.

• • •

I had slept with Mike on our first date. I had had one-night stands and mutual friends-with-benefits relationships before that. I was tired of men telling me, "I forgive you for your past," when nothing about my past had anything to do with them. I had done all sorts of things that I did not feel ashamed of, until I saw them through other people's eyes. And these men that mocked this whitefish girl, part of their behavior resulted from resentment that she didn't choose them, and part of it was envy that she had more experience than they had. If I were a man, they would ask me for advice and send me porn. But I was a woman. Therefore, they could never, ever know how experienced I was, or else I would be a whitefish, too. I still did not know what that meant, but I knew that I didn't want that word directed at me. I wish I had shamed them into silence that day. I wish I defended the whitefish girl, but I had been too afraid of them directing their attention in my direction.

So when Mike asked me to pretend to be a virgin when we met, and never speak of anything that happened in my life before he came along, of course I went along with it. It seemed the only way to keep him. I didn't understand that our subterfuge would create an uncrossable crevasse between who I was and who I thought he wanted me to be. I didn't know that trying to be someone I wasn't was not the ideal way to start a relationship.

I wanted to be a good girl. I knew how quickly crazy love can turn deranged, and I was afraid to trust my heart to lead me anywhere good. A healthy relationship, I decided, began in the head, with logical choices and compatibility of goals. I may not have had a relationship frenzied with excitement, but then again, I didn't have agony, either. Mike had a pilot's license, just like my father. He was an air traffic controller with a bachelor's degree, going to school to finish his master's, and that was sexy and impressive—not just to me, but to everyone I told. I was vicariously cool in his wake. I was a college dropout, always looking for a shortcut to success.

I did not know that he would never pilot a plane again, or that he would never finish his graduate degree. Back then, the future was filled with bright hope and pretty daydreams. We had floor plans of houses taped to our refrigerator long before we knew what state we would move to next. We made lists of all the things we would do as soon as we moved to a bigger town—things that we could not do in Key West, like eat Arby's, or go to the ballet. We were going to find at least one really good Mexican restaurant that served tacos on corn tortillas instead of flour, go to concerts and family reunions. We'd name our next cat Arugula and get a yellow Labrador retriever named Zulu Time. Then we'd buy a bulldog and name her Bougainvillea—Bogie for short. We had names picked out for a baby girl and a baby boy long before we tried to conceive them.

The first night I spent at Mike's house we slept in a tangled heap of arms and legs, like a pile of pick-up sticks. By the third night, though, he had moved to the other side of the bed, and there he remained for the rest of our relationship. He needed sleep. I needed touch, but I understood that my need for closeness wasn't as important as his need for rest. He was an air traffic controller, after all. He held many lives in his hands—more in any given day than a surgeon, or so the rhetoric went. I was in awe of him, and acquiescence became my natural state. I didn't realize on that third night all that I would lose by reluctantly moving to the other side of the bed.

I liked our brand-new, shiny apartment that was identical to the other sixty units in the complex. I loved our clean white walls, devoid of art, and the beige living-room furniture we bought together. I still had boxes of all of my precious knickknacks and dolls in the guest room closet, and I looked

forward to someday having a house in which I could display them—I didn't
know then that although we would live in five more apartments and own
three different houses, he and I would never live in a place where my sentimental flotsam would be considered appropriate.

He was my favorite person, even if I wasn't batshit nuts over him. The
I-will-die-without-you experience almost killed me the first time around,
and I felt mostly sure that what I gained in stability would more than make
up for the fire that we lacked. Besides, all the relationship books said that
lovesick fervor died down pretty quickly anyway, so if you expect to succeed
in a relationship, you had better be sure that there was substance underneath. I wanted to be a bride. My parents loved him, he got along with my
brother, and his family accepted me as well. Mike was one of five siblings
and his mother was one of six, so he provided all of the cousins and aunts
and uncles that I had never had. Unlike my first marriage, Mom and Pat
approved of this union, although Pat pulled me into the garage after dinner one night to ask, "Do you really love him? Are you sure he's interesting
enough—not too boring? I'm just worried he's too much of a homebody for
you." I reassured her that Mike was plenty interesting, and besides, I was
done with drama. I'm not sure I convinced either one of us, but I wanted it
to be true so damn badly.

Drag Fish

I bought a Christmas ornament, a fish with red glittery lips that reminded me of the drag queens I adored at the 801 Bar in Key West. My lesbian parents took me to the 801 for bingo every Sunday, and my brother introduced me to my first drag show there. From then on, every man I was serious about had to pass the 801 comfort test—if they wouldn't go, I wouldn't date them.

I had looked at the fish ornament through the store window for months on my lunch break, and even though I knew it was a foolish thing to want so badly, I finally bought the drag queen fish after the Christmas season was over. I strung rainbow-colored beads to make a chain and hung my fish from the rearview mirror of my car. For the next two years I drove around Key West with the sun sparkling on that fish's big lips, and it made me happy every day.

Mike was hired by the FAA. Even though he did not yet have a start date, he left the navy and we left Key West. We packed up our apartment and sold his car so that we could make the twenty-eight-hour drive north in one vehicle. I felt wistful about leaving my island, but I couldn't wait for the white-picket-fence life waiting for us in suburbia.

Mike and I were in the covered car park, trying to cram our life into the trunk of my Toyota Echo. I was going to miss the ocean breeze like I would miss a friend. I had sworn that I would never move north again— I had donated all my sweaters and coats to the Salvation Army years ago—but love and family were the only goals I had.

I would get to be a stay-at-home mother, now. I'd finally have the life I'd dreamed of since I was a child.

• • •

"You are taking that fish down, aren't you? I'm not driving off the island in a car with a drag queen fish hanging from the rearview mirror," Mike said. I was shocked into silence—I didn't even know how to close my half-opened mouth. All the happy bits of me crumbled like a fistful of dried leaves. I thought that he loved my quirkiness. I didn't know why he was suddenly embarrassed. I wordlessly took my fish down and packed it away. I tried not to think of who I was supposed be now that I was returning to the continental United States—what parts of me would need to join the fish in that shoebox as no longer appropriate. I had already quit my job and we had given up the apartment—it was too late to develop reservations.

I was trying very hard and earnestly not to be so much *me* anymore. I wanted to be neat and tidy and restrained. I stopped kissing girls and going to gay bars. I grew out my short, spiky hair until it was long and ordinary, and stopped streaking it surfer blond. I was happy to finally fit in—it was all I had ever wanted. Me, the daughter of a lesbian mother and a father living in far-off Alaska who no one entirely believed existed. I grew up with bad hair and braces and knowing too many answers in class. Marrying Mike would blur out who I used to be—help me finally be just like everyone else. I did not realize that "commonplace" was not something I was capable of maintaining. Nor was it something worth aspiring to become. This was what Mike wanted more than anything—to take his place in the family as a fully formed adult, well equipped with matching china and sturdy plans for the future. Perhaps I was a means to an end for him as well.

• • •

Mike and I moved to Kansas for a temporary job while we waited for the FAA's hiring freeze to lift. He was told to seek other employment for six weeks but we wound up waiting two and a half years. We were told every month to call back in another four weeks. I yearned for my island every day—I missed it like it was a person. My bones ached for home.

As a newlywed of two months, I counted fifty-seven days since we last made love. I told myself it didn't matter—sex was trivial, unimportant. I worried that there was something wrong with my craving it so much, perhaps something inherited from my father.

Warning Signs Are for Wimps

The puppy should have been a sign to give in and go back home. Zulu Time was a nearly white polar bear–looking yellow lab puppy, adorable and fluffy and about eight thousand times more work than either of us anticipated. After a week, we gave him back to the breeder. It was the first time I saw Mike cry. We wrapped our arms around each other at the side of the road and sobbed. After a few days we went back and retrieved the puppy.

The dog got up every few hours all night long. We both worked full-time jobs, so we alternated who would let the dog out at 2:00 a.m. Since we lived in an apartment, letting out the dog required pants. I traded my satin nightgowns for sweats. When it was Mike's turn to walk the dog, he pulled a pillow over his head and ignored the barking. If he waited long enough, I'd always get up and take care of the dog for him. One night I was up listening to my husband's awake-sounding breathing as the puppy barked and whined in his cage at the foot of our bed. I was tired of being the one to always give in. I kicked Mike under the covers. Hard. He got up and took care of the dog, and I went back to sleep.

The next morning, we had the biggest fight of our marriage—even bigger than any fights we had when we broke up.

"I can't believe you resorted to physical abuse," he said, or something along those lines. He denied that he was awake and ignoring the dog.

"I must have kicked you in my sleep," I replied. I was always a good liar. He chose to believe me.

• • •

At the time, I had just turned thirty and was working an entry-level job for the United States Department of Agriculture. I desperately wanted a baby—it was the only life goal I'd ever had. I was sure everything would work out once I finally had a tiny human creature of my own. After I saw that blue plus sign on the pregnancy test, nothing else mattered. From the time I was a little girl, I had wanted to be a mother. When a job opened for my husband in Cleveland, it seemed that all of our dreams were coming true.

• • •

Childbirth changed everything. So far, I had experienced a lot of the hard side of life—my first husband's motorcycle accident, followed by a house fire and running away to Key West with just the clothes on my back—but this was somehow different. When the pain hit, I was alone in it. Mike did not leave my side for twelve hours. He changed the music when I asked. He watched the monitor and told me when I was close to the peak of pain. He did not eat or sleep or rub my arm the wrong way, but I did not feel comforted by him. I had always kept a wall between us—I never let him see my broken side. Now that I needed to lean on him, I did not know how.

None of that mattered once our son was born. He had wavy brown hair and enormous blue eyes. When the doctor held him up, his tiny wrinkled face bore an expression of, "What the fuck is this?" How could we not fall head over heels for this grouchy little creature?

The second night we were home from the hospital the baby refused to sleep. Mike made a *yrnffh* noise as I crept past his side of the bed to go to the babe. I picked up my son's eight-pound body and turned him so I could look into his little balled-up face. "Listen, kid," I told him. "I'm all you got. It's just you and me here, and I'm out of ideas, so you're gonna have to meet me halfway." From that moment on, the baby and I were a team, and Mike was on the sidelines. I soothed the baby throughout that long night: walking up and down the stairs, rocking him in a chair, singing, even vacuuming around his crib in an effort to soothe him with the sound. I was not supposed to go up and down stairs or walk the baby up and down the hall but what could I do? I could not let him cry. Mike needed sleep.

I had been told to expect to pass tissue the size of golf balls after childbirth, but if I passed one the size of my fist I needed to call the doctor right away. The next day when I stood up, a blood clot larger than my hand slid wetly down my leg and landed on the floor. It scared me—I was doing too much. I took a mirror and saw that I had pulled out some of my stitches. What of it? I was a mother now. It was my job to do everything necessary to comfort this child. I did not think much about the part that Mike wasn't playing, not until later.

At first, parenting made my husband and me a team. We took turns diapering, we made charts of everything we could think of to track what helped the baby sleep—bath time, feedings, thermostat settings, pajamas. Mike was no good at night-waking though. He could not afford to be tired at work due to the many lives he held in his hands every day. I was only a secretary. I didn't mind nursing the baby at night in the tiny hard-backed rocking chair my grandfather had made long before I was born. I thought of all of the other mothers of newborns sitting in the dark and nursing their babies, and I did not feel alone. I had fallen into a deeper love with this little feral creature than I had known was possible, and I did not mind sacrificing sleep for him. I learned that people don't need nearly as much sleep as they think they do. I fell into a rhythm of waking and sleeping every few hours that lasted nearly two years.

The End of It All

That first year of our baby's life was the happiest Mike and I ever were as a couple, but it was all over when we bought the recliner.

For years, I had watched TV with my head in Mike's lap, his hands stroking my hair until I fell asleep. But now I needed to rock the baby, feed the baby, persuade the baby to go to sleep, so we bought an Ultrasuede rocking recliner. Officially, it was a present for me, but Mike quickly took it over. Night after night, Mike sat in the recliner, and I lay on the couch six feet away. He never stroked my hair again.

• • •

We both wanted a second child, so I started to chart my fertile days on a calendar in the kitchen. "Can't we just figure out your fertile days, and we only have to have sex then?" Mike asked me. Some months, he could not bring himself to manage that. I was silently furious—not only did I feel spurned, but I wanted a second child very badly. Still, he eventually managed to bring himself to have sex with me on a day that might be productive, and we did conceive a second child.

• • •

I had never allowed myself to dream of anything beyond becoming a wife and mother. Then I woke up one day during my second pregnancy flooded with stories, and I could not stop writing. The words came pouring out of me and I wrote every minute I could tuck in between caring for our toddler, and then lay awake in the dark beside my sleeping husband and dreamed of sentences and characters instead of family vacations and preschools. I asked Mike to read what I had written, but he wasn't interested. The second time around, pregnancy filled me with sexual hormones, and his words, "No, not now, don't you start that," left me seething.

One day I woke with a stabbing headache that made my eyes blur and my stomach rise up.

"I can't miss work," Mike told me. "I just got a warning letter for excessive absences. Can't you call one of your friends?"

I called the few friends I had in town—my parents lived several hours away—but no one could help. Our toddler and I were alone in the apartment for the ten hours Mike was gone, and I alternated between pressing my face into a facial steamer and vomiting over the toilet, while the Baby Einstein DVD played on repeat. Two days later, Mike called off work again. "I just can't do it today," he said. That's when I started to hate him.

I asked Mike to go to a special labor and delivery class. My first labor had been so painful, and I felt sure that there had to be a better way. He asked if he could just read the book instead, and then he asked me to just highlight the relevant pages so he didn't have to read the whole thing. In the end, he never read more than a few sentences. It was another resentment I could not forget.

• • •

Labor and delivery were different the second time around. My anger, which I had never spoken aloud, had eaten away all of my affection toward Mike. I hoped that childbirth would erase the bitterness that had settled into my shoulders, sternum, and the pit of my stomach. I attempted a water birth, and he climbed into the bathtub fully clothed to put pressure on my back. The doula and midwife lauded him for being an exceptional husband and father, but once again, I could not lean on him when I needed him the most—not because he wasn't there, but because I had created a shell and I could not dismantle it now when my insides were being ripped apart. Mike caught our second child and eased him out of my body. He cut the umbilical cord. But he found the pull-out couch in the hospital room too uncomfortable to sleep on, and insisted that we leave the hospital after one night, even though I had not yet showered off the residue of childbirth. I didn't know how to refuse him.

It was easy for me to think of this baby as entirely my own. Because I nursed, Mike never did a feeding. When I switched to cloth diapers, something that disgusted him, Mike no longer wiped any bottoms. Many nights, he didn't come to bed. The baby and I were alone together night after night.

One day my best friend asked if she could come over while her husband had an appointment in the neighborhood. Mike said no, because she had already been over once that week, and he didn't like visitors. I was glad I told her over the phone, so I would not see the pity and disgust in her eyes. I did not know when my husband became my father, able to tell me what I could and couldn't do, and I didn't know how to rewind back to who I used to be.

• • •

I quit my job to be a stay-at-home mother, and we relied solely on Mike's income, so when Mike made the rules, I did not argue. The children and I had to be kept safe so nothing could hurt us, but this protection restricted me to a flat, one-dimensional world. If it was raining out, Mike pleaded with me to stay home. He forbade me to take the babies to any playground that was not visible from the street. He did not want me to go walking with them in the woods in the neighborhood park. I couldn't fly, I couldn't scuba dive. I couldn't swim in the ocean or Lake Erie. I couldn't go out and I couldn't have anyone in. I could write, but only if no one knew it was me that was writing. I gave the love and he paid the bills, sitting blankly in his recliner night after night while I slept alone.

The monotony of staying home all day drove me crazy, doing nothing but wiping bottoms and noses to the soundtrack of children's television. I was tired of having no money of my own, so I decided to go back to work part-time, to save my sanity and the children. I wasn't sure all three of us would survive if I continued staying home with them all day, every day.

"I want to go back to work," I told Mike.

"You aren't allowed to work until the baby is in kindergarten," he replied. He kept looking straight ahead. "That's the deal."

I didn't say anything. My mouth couldn't form the words to stand up for myself. All my indignation rattled around inside my body, a mass of roiling discontent and an angry energy that could not get out. *We'll see,* I thought, though I said nothing. I wasn't going to stay with a man who thought he could dictate the terms of my life. Not again.

. . .

We lived as roommates. Within a few weeks after childbirth I was eager to resume sex, but Mike was completely disinterested. His constant refusal— *no, not now, don't you start that*—shredded me. I did not know then that he considered sex too dirty to have with the mother of his children. I told him my deepest sexual fantasy, and he spat on the ground.

I turned online to find readers of my stories and affirmation that I was not invisible. I started taking pictures of myself—zoomed and cropped to show cleavage, but never my face, and never naked—teasing pictures that made me feel desirable. I texted and exchanged selfies with other men, but didn't have sex with anyone. Was it cheating? It certainly wasn't proper married behavior. Realizing the injustice of showing these pictures to other men and not to my husband, I emailed Mike a picture of my leopard thong peeking out of the back of my low-rise jeans. He demanded that I never send him such a picture again.

It wasn't only physical intimacy I missed. I asked to go to the *Nutcracker*, part of my Christmas tradition from childhood. He told me, "I don't have to do that anymore, we're married now." I no longer wanted to be married to this man. Affection alone could no longer sustain me. We tried counseling, but I wasn't looking for a way to save our marriage. I wanted permission to leave it.

. . .

How could I break my children's family apart merely to pursue my own happiness? I remember standing in my pink bedroom when I was eight or nine years old, promising myself that if I ever had children, I would not get divorced, unless my husband hit me or cheated on me. I'd always remember how it felt to be a child, and I would always put my children first. I had tried so hard to blend into blue and beige, but once I achieved it, I realized all those quirky, colorful things were what made me whole. My weird wonky funkiness was what made me beautiful. If I didn't revive my best self, I would never be able to mother my children properly.

. . .

I realized that I would not make it eighteen more years until the boys were out of high school. If I were going to leave, I needed to do it now, while both of them were still in diapers, before they grew old enough to remember a life with both parents living in the same house. I'd lie awake at night and feel time ticking away—the pressure of my children's developing memory. I told myself over and over, "But he would not read the words I wrote." These words stood in for all the other words I could not say aloud, wound-words caused by both our actions and our inactions. I couldn't let my dreams fade, growing a little fainter every year until they vanished. I did not want my boys to become blank faces staring into a television set next to their father, too afraid to go out and play, uninspired by a mother who drained all the color out of herself in an effort to fit in.

I lived in words and dreamed on pages, my once-starved passion now robust and hungry. Run-on sentences devoured the empty space on my com- 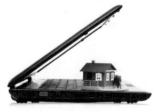 puter screen night after night. This dream life hovered at the tip of my fingers, if only I could dive into who I longed to be. I wrote my yearn- ing into hundreds of pages of romantic stories and trusted the words would carry me back to the self I had abandoned, the one that I had hidden from the light for the past seven years.

. . .

I dreamed over and over again of a house I didn't own—an old colonial, quirky and full of charm. It had hardwood floors that didn't need refinish- ing and I covered them with Oriental rugs and funky area rugs. There was thick solid-wood trim and heavy oak doors. I would paint the dining room aubergine—no, not that dark, but a little redder than plum—more exactly the color of the sky when the sunset fades into the ocean. In my dream I would paint my bedroom orange, or sometimes it was my kitchen that was tangerine or burnished copper, glazed so that brushstrokes were visible. I dreamed of cupboards filled with Fiestaware that I had never owned. The rooms in my dream house were no longer exactly square but that was okay—the long hallway would be perfect for racing Matchbox cars and sliding around in socks.

I had a lover, too, in these dreams, with thick, dark hair. He was smart and we laughed a lot, and we painted the whole house together in paint-splattered, well-worn jeans before we moved in, and we danced barefoot in the empty house. We held hands often and walked in the rain. He made me get off the couch and do something, I made him lounge around the house on a Saturday afternoon. Our clothes were old and our dishes chipped but that made them softer and better, because we didn't have to worry too much about breaking them. I sewed beads onto everything and covered the couch with too many throw pillows that I made myself, and I tossed them at my lover when we argued over movies and how they should have ended. We had a piano that the cat walked across in the middle of the night and cracks in the plaster ceiling we meant to fix but never cared enough to bother with. We made love for hours on crisp white linens. We had parties and let the kids stay up late to watch TV in our bedroom while we laughed and played music and drank wine, and there were never enough chairs for people so I just sat on the floor.

I told myself this was a sappy, naive dream, but it kept reappearing, no matter how hard I tried to squelch it. There was no room for Mike in my dream house, not only because he wasn't my dream man, but because his dreams were of new construction—pressboard cabinets, linoleum floors and Berber carpeting. I could not sacrifice the life I wanted in order to keep the life I had. I didn't know how to resolve it. Depression settled in to my bones, my muscles, my hair follicles. Mike sat at the foot of the recliner as I sobbed. I had no words for what was wrong—not that I could tell him in a way that made sense. He vowed to do anything he could to help me feel better. I longed to throw myself under a bus. If you have felt sadness and despair so deep that you long for gravel under your face and tire rubber crushing you, then you understand that there are other problems besides adultery or abuse that are irreconcilable.

If I died, my children's lives would be simpler. They wouldn't be torn between two houses. They would grow up just having a daddy, their mother dead before they could remember her. In the end, I decided they'd be happier with divorced parents than no mother—that leaving actually was a form of putting the children first. We would just have to make parenting work from two houses.

• • •

The word *passion* derives from the Latin *patere*: to suffer. But to fulfill my passion, it was Mike who had to suffer the most. I dismantled his dreams and abandoned his life like they were detritus after a parade: old candy wrappers and red plastic cups mixing with pebbles and cigarette butts at the edge of the road. The truth was, though, that I never was who he needed, either. He longed for long fingernails, and mine were bitten to the quick. The ultimate irony—you cast your pearls before swine, and the boar says he prefers rhinestones.

• • •

Mike told me, "You weren't crazy until after you left me." He was wrong— I had been crazy all along but I starved and denied and hid the crazy that made me beautiful: the part of me that loved orange sneakers and glitter, my urge to dance on sidewalks and speak in funny accents at restaurants, my love of inappropriate conversations and the way parades always made me cry—the part of me that was wounded and fragile, and that desperately needed to live in the light.

I needed a climactic moment to allow myself to escape this life, but neither Mike nor I would instigate one. We both avoided conflict, carefully smiling and stepping around each other in our bland, beige house. We discussed the children, the dogs, his job, but we both refused to talk about anything that mattered. I slowly vanished, going to my mother's every weekend with the children, lying on my parents' living-room rug and begging my parents to tell me what to do, while my toddler played with his toy cars nearby and the baby struggled to push his little round belly up off the carpet and hold himself up with his chubby little arms.

"Have an affair," my mother told me.

"Leave him," Pat said, "and I will make sure you and the children are okay."

One day when Mike went to work, I wanted to pull my veins out of my skin, tear out my hair, hit the walls and scream, "Look at me—I'm not just a mother, I'm still a sexual being! I'm still an adult with dreams and needs of her own." That day, instead of retreating to my online world of friends and stories, I emptied the children's dresser drawers, packed up the car, and drove to my parents' house.

"Please, Lara, you have to wait and tell him after he gets home from work," my mother admonished me, but I couldn't say the words to his face. Over the phone, I told my husband, "I can't do this anymore, I have to go." It took him four days to understand that "I have to go" meant "forever," not a weekend visit at my parents' house.

"Not seeing my children every day is a death sentence," he told me. Still, I did not go back.

When we were married, Mike refused to watch both boys at the same time, insisting that I drag either a newborn or a toddler to the grocery store—even in the cold, even in the rain. When I left him and he insisted on keeping the boys overnight three nights of every week, I was astonished. I do not know if I could have left if I had known. I thought in leaving I would make the boys more mine—I wound up making them less. That first year, everyone told me to wait it out—my parents, my lawyer, my boss— that Mike would tire of taking the children, especially when he had to drive them a half an hour to school in the mornings. Cleveland rush hour was guaranteed to wear him down and I would have the children all the time.

In the end, the traffic wasn't enough to break my ex-husband. It turned out that he was a much better single father than he had ever been when we were married. I had to accept that I was not keeping my boys full-time, and realize that although it was devastating for me, it was best for them to have both parents in their lives. I created this split family dynamic, and now we all had to live with it.

PART TWO
BECOMING ONLY MAMA

Preparing the Reader for the Ensuing Chaos: How to Make a Light Whiskey Sour

I didn't drink alcohol at all from the time I was fifteen until I was twenty-six. I was a little late to learn about things like the important ratio of food to alcohol, but I eventually gained that knowledge as most people do—the hard and embarrassing way involving kneeling in front of a toilet while moaning. However, I did learn most of these important lessons well before I got pregnant. Of course, I couldn't drink while pregnant, and couldn't drink much while nursing, so it was several years before alcohol came back into my life.

As a single mother, I mostly drank wine, though I had other beverages in the house for friends. Once, I ran out of wine and filled my glass up with whiskey, and I am here to say that there is a very big difference between a glass of pinot grigio and a glass of Jack Daniel's, even though they aren't horribly different in color. The difference is mainly detectable in terms of emotional response to things like tiny duckie slippers found when the children are at their father's, or sad abandoned dog commercials set to music by Sarah McLachlan, and the urge to write melodramatic poetry. I needed a lighter drink for when I ran out of wine and only had whiskey and also didn't want to cry or write bad poetry, so I learned to make a whiskey sour. Although I like to drink alcohol, I don't like the calories or to get really drunk, so I make a weaker whiskey sour than most people. Probably all people.

Light Whiskey Sour

Disclaimer: light does not refer to calories, but rather lighter on the alcohol as compared to a wineglass full of whiskey. How much you pour determines the alcohol content.

Ingredients
Simple syrup (Recipe below. Don't be scared, it's really easy.)
Whiskey (I use Jack Daniel's)
Lemon juice
Club soda/flavored seltzer/something that tastes *blah* and has no calories. Not the artificially sweetened seltzer-type drinks.

Procedure
1. Make simple syrup:
    OK, this is going to sound like a whole lot of work, but it's not, I promise. I avoid doing things that are a lot of work, and this is one of those things that is way easier to make than to try and find in a store, at least unless you already know where to buy simple syrup—I obviously do not.

    First off, the next time you run out of spaghetti sauce, olives, or pickles, instead of recycling the jar, wash it and save the lid. You will need it. You actually don't need a large jar, just something that holds about a cup or two of liquid.

    Pour one cup of water and one cup of sugar into a pot and bring to a boil. Stir until dissolved. That's

(continued)

it. Nothing too complicated. Once it boils, pour into the clean jar you liberated from the recycling bin. It doesn't even need to be refrigerated. See? Not scary. You conquered simple syrup!

Side note: I once ran out of simple syrup but had some homemade hummingbird food. To make hummingbird food, you dissolve ¼ cup sugar in 1 cup boiling water, then add some red food coloring. It not only tasted fine, but it made the drink a pretty color. It also has fewer calories.

2. The rest of the drink:
Fill a full-sized glass with ice (not a short mixed-drink tumbler, but like a regular one you drink water out of). Put three of your fingers around the bottom, and pour the whiskey to the top of your fingers. Move your hand up, and place two fingers on the top line of the whiskey (on the outside of the glass, obviously), and pour lemon juice to the top of your fingers again.

(Note: if you don't have lemon juice but do have lime juice and wonder if it is close enough, it's not really. You might think lime is really just a green lemon-cousin, but apparently it needs to be yellow to work correctly.)

Returning to the recipe: Place one finger on the top of the liquid line and pour simple syrup up to that line. Fill the rest of the glass with club soda or whatever bland and tasteless seltzer you have. Stir with a knife. Why a knife? I don't know, but it goes all the way down to the bottom of the glass, which seems most efficient. I take the rest of the can of seltzer/club soda with me to the table and refill as I drink, without adding more whiskey because I don't want

the alcohol or the calories but I like the taste. Note:
real bartenders add a dash of egg white to this drink,
but I have no idea what magic that adds, and salmonella scares me, so I don't do it.

Now that you are properly prepared, I return you to our story, already
in progress.

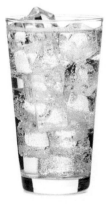

It's a Nice Life, but Someone's Got to Pay for It

I left my husband when my youngest was four months old—just before my eldest's third birthday. A couple from church asked me to house-sit, and then they let me stay until I found a place of my own. Their adult daughter, Asterisk, was also going through a divorce, and she moved in with her parents the same week I did. Asterisk's youngest son was four years old, and he and my eldest quickly became buddies. Asterisk and I house-hunted the same month and moved into our new single-mama homes within a week of each other. We went to Target together and bought pans and vacuum cleaners and everything else we needed but had left behind.

It was Asterisk and her family who greeted me after my first day of work. I called Asterisk's mother every time I missed my exit on the way to or from my job and wound up on the wrong side of town. Asterisk even supplied friends to help us both move.

• • •

I found a job on Craigslist. It paid less money than I had made in a decade, offered no insurance or paid days off, and wasn't full-time, yet I loved it. We designed collegiate sports apparel—mostly socks and baseball hats. I did the graphic design more or less adequately and the bookkeeping extremely well. I got to have grown-up conversations and lose myself in projects that didn't involve finger paint. I felt capable, smart, and funny for the first time in a very long time. I made a decision not to bring my personal life into the office—for the first time ever—and work became a refuge even on the worst days.

I picked up a second job at my church as the Director of Religious Education. Except for Sundays and the occasional evening meeting, I could work at home, and between the two jobs I got by. My parents bought a house in a nice suburb and rented it to me for far below the going rate. Without them, I could have only afforded a two-bedroom apartment in subsidized housing. When the divorce was finalized, my bank made me refinance my car loan to remove my ex-husband, and since I had not been at my house or job for very long, they were going to double my interest rate. My parents stepped in again and assumed the loan on the family minivan, charging me the same payment as I had been paying before. Although I was poor, I was "privileged-poor." I hadn't kept that promise I made myself back in childhood to never get divorced, but I got to stay home with my children most of the time—I needed childcare only one and a half days a week. This is not to say that I had a lot of money. If I didn't use cloth diapers and instead bought Pampers each week I wouldn't have made it, even with my parents providing me a house at incredibly low rent. My stepmother had negotiated to buy the house "as-is" and insisted that all the items in the house remain after the sale. The house had sat empty for several years, but the Realtor staged it to avoid listing it as vacant, so there were a few sheets and towels, a stack of dishes, an old sewing machine in the basement, and miscellaneous tools stored in the built-in workbench in the basement.

I found a 12 x 12 pillow sham neatly folded on the closet shelf, and dyed it from pale pink to coral. It was one of a very few decorative items I had. I never would've spent good money to buy a decorative pillow, not then, when I was struggling to pay off old debt and buy new clothes for growing boys. If anything was left over, it went to savings, not to frivolous things, but like so many other things I needed, it came with the house. On the rare occasions that I actually made my bed, the small throw pillow sat as reassurance that the life I had always wanted was at hand. It was as if the house knew I needed that smile as much as I needed the leftover tools in the basement.

When I first moved in I gave *Came with the House* tours to anyone who came over, pointing out the futon, baker's rack, and microwave like a tour guide. Asterisk's school-aged children became my docents and recited along with me on playdates. We showed off the nonmotorized push mower with a dull blade, the large stacks of plates and dishes with colorful flowers painted around their edges, the floor lamp in the living room, the metal chairs on the front porch. All of these once-loved items eased my transition from married to single; they protected me from the void of what I left behind. Everything I needed that I hadn't gotten around to buying could be found in the closets. A drain snake, rusty but functional, saved me from a plumber's bill. I found a case of light bulbs, two Swiffers, and rolls of clear tape. I hung up the curtains I found on closet shelves and used old pink towels that were just a little bit unraveled at the edges.

I wanted to write to the former owner and thank her. Like me, she had been a single mother. Like me, she had two boys and a dog. Eventually she fell in love, got married, and moved away. There was hope for me, too. She left behind pieces to guide me on the road behind her. She even left cleaning supplies and enough toilet paper to last me that first year, when all I could focus on was changing diapers and getting to work on time.

• • •

I made the decision to apply for WIC—a government assistance program for women, infants, and children. It requires participants to qualify both financially and nutritionally. You can't just be poor—you have to be poor *and* failing to feed your children adequately. It's devastatingly hard to apply

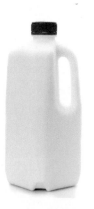

for such a program. It was embarrassing and degrading and still my best option. I was lucky that the local office was staffed by several very nice women who helped me with the forms—left to my own devices, I would have given up. Nutritionally, the only need they could find was that I gave my toddler too much milk. Every month I went in to get my coupons, I had to sit through a counseling session where they showed me plastic cups in various sizes and discussed how much milk a three-year-old actually needed, versus how much milk I was routinely giving him. Sometimes the social worker apologized for having to go through the demo and complimented me on being a good mother, and sometimes the social worker was very stern with me about my over-milking.

I was given one coupon for all the items I was allowed each month. One pound of full-fat cheese, one box of preapproved cereal, one bottle of very specific juice. The coupon was all or nothing, so if I got the wrong juice, I either had to hold up the line while I went back to retrieve the correct juice, or I had to forgo the free juice. I always chose to forgo the juice and tried not to cry. As much as people hate to stand in line behind someone with coupons, it is just as bad to be the one who is using them, knowing everyone is impatient and that you are holding them up.

I only stuck with WIC for a few months. The benefit—around $80–$100 a month—was helpful, but I easily made up for it when gas prices went down. I got a raise at my day job, then another one. I was managing to provide the life I wanted, as long as I didn't give in to the longing for too many worldly possessions.

ONLY MAMA

HOME | POSTS | ABOUT THIS BLOG | ABOUT ME

Divorce Is Just Weird Sometimes— An Ode to a Dancing Gopher

When my ex and I split up, we didn't fight over the big things. We agreed easily over the division of all the major assets: property, furniture, pets. Where we got stuck was the little things. We honestly argued over who got to keep the broom (I lost).

We managed to come to a shared parenting agreement fairly easily, and I have few regrets over how we handled our dissolution except for one thing: the dancing gopher. I gave in on the dancing gopher, and I still regret it to this day.

Once upon a time, I had a dear bestest friend named Jesse, who also happened to be a drag queen. We were both recovering from bad relationships and lived together for nearly a year. One day we went to a bar. Jesse was underage, so it must have been a bar/restaurant. All I know is that I ate black beans and rice. That is not relevant at all. It's also not particularly interesting, but I thought I'd mention it to make my story longer and filled with solid details.

At the bar was a man, and that man had a dancing gopher. A fabulous, fuzzy, adorable gopher that shook his fuzzy little bottom and danced to the *Caddyshack* theme song.

The gopher was the most wonderful thing Jesse or I could imagine, and when we learned that he could be had for a bargain price at the local Walgreens—let's be honest, a dancing gopher at *any* price is a bargain—Jesse or I, or both of us, raced down to

Walgreens and bought one. (The detail of who bought the gopher is much more relevant than the fact that I ate black beans and rice, but sadly I have forgotten it. Now you see why I included the less relevant factoid.)

The gopher was perfect and brought nothing but pure joy but somehow looked, well, naked. Luckily, we had been given a bag of broken and mismatched jewelry someone thought we could make crafts with, and we quickly accessorized our fuzzy dancing friend with earrings, a necklace, and a flower lei. He was even more fabulous now, and we showed him off to every visitor to our humble abode.

Eventually Jesse left town, and I got custody of the gopher. I brought him with me when I, too, moved away. I cherished him for years, dragging him from house to house and state to state, always keeping him in a place of honor in the living room. He still sang, but after a few years he no longer shook his fuzzy little moneymaker. Eventually he would end up on a shelf in the family room of my old marital home.

I was surprised in the property settlement that he became a creature of contention. He was mine. I brought him into the marriage, and I planned on bringing him back out. Ex-Mr. Only-Mama insisted that *he* should keep him, though, because he loved the movie *Caddyshack* more than I did, and besides, the dancing gopher really belonged to the children now, and belonged in their playroom. I gave in and left my beloved dancing gopher there.

The last time I was at my ex's house, the dancing gopher was still displayed in his place of honor, though stripped of all his drag queen finery. I pushed his little button, and saw that his batteries had run down or his mechanism had worn out. Regardless, he no longer sang or danced.

(continued)

Still, though, maybe it's good that he's there. In a house totally stripped of anything else *Mama*, he alone is proof that I once lived there. He alone watches over my children when I am away.

. . . .

Posted by Lara L Monday, October 28, 2013 at 7:04 PM
Labels: Not My Finer Moments, Single Parenting

Negotiating with Spiders

Our house was small and perfect. The living room was light blue, the kitchen was orange, and my bedroom was pink. It had a second-floor balcony and most amazing of all—the ability to turn on the living-room light from the second floor. This meant that any time I heard a scary noise, I flipped the light switch and waited for any robbers to vacate the premises before I went downstairs to investigate. It must have worked—I never encountered a scary burglar after hearing a thud in the night.

I nursed my baby and tried to get my toddler to eat and we slept all three of us in my double bed. I never slept more than two consecutive hours when the children were home. I fought to form a new life for myself, one with friends and art and love. I dated poorly, but with determination. A relationship was high on my list of things to accomplish, and I figured I could cross it off in six months to a year. Guilt lived liquid in the marrow of my bones—regret for not being a person who could be satisfied with the mundane, but not regret for what I had done. Loneliness ransacked the house when the children were with their father—churning and dissolving every atom of air. It always surprised me that the furniture wasn't overturned by it. I dropped to the floor holding one small baby sock in my hands.

I wrote long hours into the night and could not stop. I made collages out of scraps from magazines and hung them on my walls. I attended a weeklong writing workshop and enrolled in college, because finishing my bachelor's degree was right up there on my list of priorities just behind finding a new man. I sat in class with eighteen-year-olds and did my homework on the front porch in the winter air. It was freezing outside; the sharp wind was biting and desolate, but it brought life to my body after living numbed for so long.

There was exhilaration in my newfound freedom. I could wear mismatched socks and sparkly sneakers. I could swim in Lake Erie, go to Africa, hang glide, or do any one of the numerous things my ex-husband didn't approve of. I could eat corn chips for dinner and let the children stay in pajamas all day. The previous owner of my house had left a wall-mounted CD player in the bathroom. I played the same CD every morning when the boys were at their father's house, one I had made myself with just one song on it, repeated over and over: "Killing in the Name" by Rage Against the Machine. "Fuck you I won't do what you tell me . . ." I screamed along with the lyrics as the soapy water ran through my hair and pooled by my fire-engine-red toenails. This was the self I was proudest of—I wanted to be braver, less well-behaved, more *me* in the face of society. I had always allowed myself to be swallowed by this notion of being a good girl, and it was asphyxiating me. "And now you do what they told ya, now you're under control . . ." I was done with doing what they told me. Trying to fit in and tone down my peculiarity had flatted me out to a one-dimensional person devoid of passion or humor. I screamed along with the song, spitting out the shampoo that ran into my mouth. The truth was, I didn't know how to fight for myself, how to hold on to who I was in relationships, but I knew I needed to learn.

• • •

I had never lived completely on my own before, without a boyfriend, husband, or roommate. Yes, technically I wasn't "alone," as someone pointed out once—I had the children five days a week, but toddlers are more like badly behaved pets than life partners or even roommates. I had to learn to fully rely on myself and, let's be honest, finally grow all the way up. I was a mother of two small people. I had already been the one to do all the diapering and feeding of the children, but now I had to mow the lawn, take out the garbage, and all the other tasks that heretofore had fallen to my ex-husband.

The first heavy snowfall found me unprepared. Luckily, my house's previous owner left an old metal shovel with a slightly bent scoop in the garage. I had no heavy gloves, so I wore my brand-new orange oven mitts as I cleared the driveway. When my car refused to start on Christmas Eve, I jumped the battery myself while wearing high heels and my church dress.

One night after the children were asleep, I was watching television in bed when the house suddenly went dark. It was either from a rapist/murderer who cut the power to aid in his attack, or the space heater had tripped the circuit breaker yet again. In the quiet blackness, it was really a toss-up which felt more likely. I owned several flashlights, but I had foolishly allowed the boys to play with them and I had no idea where they were. I crept downstairs using my cell phone as a flashlight, trying not to think of potential psycho killers waiting downstairs. It was up to me to protect the house, even if doing so scared me in small, foolish ways. After I flipped the breakers and restored the light, the adrenaline rush filled me with glee like a proud ten-year-old child.

• • •

I have been afraid of spiders for as long as I can remember. In fact, at my job interview I told my boss that I would happily pick up his dry cleaning, but that I would never under any circumstances take responsibility for killing/removing any bugs. But when the boys and I moved into our cheerful new house, I realized it would be inappropriate to expect a three-year-old child to man up and squish bugs for me. Our house was funky and hip and eighty-plus years old, and I had to admit that the spiders had established squatters' rights to the place. Also, there were a whole lot more of them than there were of me, and if I angered them, they could swarm me in my sleep and also possibly eat the baby.

I made a deal with them: any spider smaller than a nickel would be allowed to stay unmolested. Spiders larger than a nickel but smaller than a quarter would be nervously relocated to the out-of-doors. But any spider larger than a quarter would be destroyed by any means necessary. High-heeled shoe. Vacuum cleaner. Napalm.

The spider contract worked out well for six years. Only twice did I find spiders larger than a quarter dangling over my bed waiting to kill me as I slept. (Probably by dropping into my open mouth, having babies inside me, and exploding out through my nasal cavity.) And technically I only killed one once, with a shoe. The other I vacuumed while standing on the bed, one arm extending the wand, drenched in cold sweat. It presumably lived and escaped to live a happy life somewhere else in the ~~house~~ neighborhood.

I was getting by as the sole defender of the house. In terms of potential intruders of the two-legged variety, various friends kept promising to give me a wooden baseball bat, and they kept forgetting. A friend, Herman, gave me a plastic Wiffle ball bat, which he found hysterical. He was lucky that it didn't fit up either of his nostrils. For a long time, I had a large empty wine bottle under the bed—not the regular size, but the big-girl double capacity variety, along with a claw hammer with only one claw that the previous homeowner had left in the basement. But I had a secret weapon— my neighbors.

For the first time in my life, I knew the people not only on either side of my house, but directly across the street and on the diagonals as well. My next-door neighbor had a teenaged daughter who babysat. Across the street was a single father who played acoustic guitar on his front step. Yes, one neighbor's cigar smoke occasionally wafted into my open windows, but I trusted that if someone came to kill us in the middle of the night, Gino would intercede or at least call the police. For the first time, I felt safe when I was alone. My neighborhood held me and the boys in the palm of its hand. And five years later, when Tiny Pants rode a two-wheeler without training wheels for the first time, yelling, "I'm only five years old!" at the top of his lungs, the nameless neighbors who had watched us walk to the park at the end of the street week after week stood up on their porches and cheered for Tiny.

When I decided to trust the universe to protect me, I stopped being afraid. I didn't even mind being home alone at night when the children were at their father's. As long as the spiders were smaller than a quarter, obviously.

Introducing the Stars of Our Show: Big Pants and Tiny Pants

Memoir is a hard beast for family to live with; just ask my mother. At the very beginning of my writing career I sat in a memoir workshop and listened to writers argue about the ethics of writing about children. Yet, raising children has been the single most important thing in my life. Not writing about it seemed to nullify its significance. Children matter, and parenting matters, and mothers are still women with needs of their own. This book, for me, is a love song to my children and my younger, more awkward self. But to write about my children, I needed to give them plausible deniability. The boys and I have different last names, but I wanted to go one step further into obscurity, so I refer to my boys as Big Pants and Tiny Pants. Tiny Pants likes to be called Tiny Pants in real life (he is currently ten) and Big Pants, at twelve, absolutely hates to be called Big Pants, but he gave me permission to use the alias in the book. He's old enough to appreciate anonymity.

When we moved out of the family home, Tiny Pants was four months old. He was a happy, chubby, nearly bald, blue-eyed baby. He inherited my father's ears, which stuck out in a rather elfin fashion. Big Pants was just shy of three years old, and his hair, which had been dark at birth, had grown lighter as he aged, so now he was platinum blond. When I was pregnant with my first child, I carefully explained to Mike, hereafter referred to as

Daddy Pants, that he had to accept that the baby would most likely look like me. I have brown eyes and had dark brown hair (which has amazingly turned blond as I aged, instead of gray). I explained to Daddy Pants patiently and sweetly that my genes were going to decimate his blue-eyed red-haired recessive gene pool. He said he understood. However, the universe laughed at me and gave me a beautiful blue-eyed blond-haired son. Twice. In black-and-white photos, Big Pants looks exactly like I did as a baby, but unfortunately, the real world is in Technicolor, so everywhere we went, I heard variations of, "I bet you look just like your daddy! You must be Daddy's boy!" and other similar annoyances. One day, a well-meaning relative was holding Big Pants and crooned, "You have Jake's eyes!" Jake was Daddy's six-year-old first cousin, once removed. I channeled that green-vomiting, head-spinning girl in *The Exorcist* and yelled, "He has my eyes and his father's coloring!"

Tiny Pants had blue eyes that were not quite the same as but similar to his brother's, but he had almost no hair at all. What hair he did have formed a point in the middle of his forehead, like Eddie on *The Munsters*. Tiny Pants was always smiling and laughing at his older brother like a happy potato, his snuggly chubbiness made even rounder by the large cloth diapers he wore. I called him my "puppy baby," because he was always chewing and drooling on everything, and his default expression was widemouthed glee, like a bald Labrador retriever.

I was an indulgent parent. I couldn't bear to hear my babies cry. Big Pants hated to sleep, and the only way I knew to get him to go to sleep was to hold him and dance to the *80s Dance Mix* CD I bought off an infomercial five years before. I held his head against my sternum with one hand, the other arm supporting his body, and his arms hung around my neck. "Video Killed the Radio Star" was first. I sang and spun, I did front kicks and side lunges. He got drowsy. By the time the third track, "Hungry Like the Wolf," was over, he was fast asleep, his arms and legs hanging limp by my sides. Sometimes I kept dancing for another song, reveling in the warm love of my toddler and the nostalgia of the music. And other times I'd turn off the song a minute too soon, he'd wake up, and I'd have to restart the CD and go through it all over again. It was generally when I needed him to sleep the most that he was unable to—perhaps there was a tension in my body he could feel. Once asleep, I carried him upstairs and laid him in his wooden toddler bed. I knew he'd only last a few hours in his own bed, then would sneak in beside me in the middle of the night, just like his baby brother, who started the night asleep in his Pack 'n Play at the foot of my bed, but always wound up in the double bed with me. They slept next to me or on top of me, and I carried them both everywhere we went—one child in each arm.

Big Pants hadn't cared much for being a baby. He wanted to be held all the time, and if I sat him down, he would make this unhappy growling complaint that sounded like he had a motor in him, a closed-mouth *mrrrrrr*. It wasn't until he was able to roll around and get himself where he wanted to go that he became a happy baby. So in those early days, I sang to him all the time. I tried "Gypsy Rover," my brother's favorite song when we were little. I tried show tunes and my favorite childhood song, "Anathea." Nothing worked until I sang "Hava Nagila" one day and he instantly quieted. I don't know if it was the novelty of the Hebrew words or the fact that it was the only song I could sing on tune that did it, but if I sang it low and slow, he'd fall asleep. That became his song throughout his toddlerhood—when he was sick, or scared, or when everything else I tried to get him to sleep failed.

• • •

Big Pants had wanted a sibling very badly, so when Tiny Pants cried, I told Big Pants, "You were the one who wanted a brother, so now we have to deal with him." I meant to keep him from being resentful—it was like getting a puppy. Tiny Pants had a baby song, too, "Sea of Love." If I was out of the room and he started crying, Big Pants would sing to his brother for me in his little two-year-old voice, "Do you wemembah, when we met . . ." and Tiny's tears ceased.

• • •

The boys were always close, and I wondered if the divorce made them closer still. After all, they were the most constant person in each other's lives—the only family member they saw every single day. When I took them to the planetarium for the first time, Tiny Pants, at two years old, was scared of the dark. He pulled away from me and sat in his brother's chair until the show was over. How much had the divorce hurt my babies? Was it as hard for them to be away from me as it was for me to be away from them? When they were gone I kept myself busy: taking classes, going out to eat, working late—anything to reduce the time I spent alone in the house without them. If I didn't put away their toys the first hour after they left, every time I saw them I became overwhelmed with grief, and then was unable to clean up at all. But I tried not to show it. I didn't want the kids to feel torn between their parents, or feel guilty for having fun without me.

When I left their father, both boys had their own rooms, and I set up my new house with a crib in one bedroom and a toddler bed in the other. Daddy Pants decided to have the boys share a room at his house after I moved out, so when I tried to put them down in their own rooms, the boys wanted nothing to do with it. "Tiny!" Big Pants cried, standing at the baby gate at the doorway of his room. "Big!" Tiny Pants echoed as he stood in his crib. I gave up and put them both in the same room, but the finished attic was the only room large enough to fit two beds and a couple of dressers. Luckily, my father had made a wooden fence with a gate at the top of the attic stairs, and it became their habitat, filled with sunlight and toys and enough room for a pop-up firehouse tent.

In Which Big Pants and I Accidentally Misplace the Baby

During the six weeks we lived with Asterisk's parents, Tiny Pants started sort-of crawling. He pulled himself up onto all fours and rocked back and forth, mouth agape in a very adorable and droolly expression of wonder, then plopped back onto his belly on the rug. It was very exciting but not anything close to locomotion. Since he wasn't mobile when we moved into our new home, I could still set Tiny Pants on a blanket on the floor and go into the kitchen and come back with a reasonable expectation that he would still be more or less where we had left him.

One day, Big Pants (still in diapers himself, and only big by comparison) wanted a snack, so we left Tiny Pants on his blanket per usual and walked ten steps into the kitchen. The house was perfect and colorful and quaint but also really small, so it was pretty easy to keep an eye on everyone and get snacks most of the time. On this particular day, though, we returned from our sojourn to the cabinet of all that was holy and good (by which I mean carbs, of course) and discovered that the baby was missing.

A missing baby is a cause for extreme panic, even when the front door is locked, because babies are not supposed to go missing under any circumstances, especially when you are new to this single-mother thing and not entirely sure you are up to the task. Besides, like puppies, babies fit in lots of places, chew on everything they see, and don't come when they're

called. Big Pants and I looked under the table, behind the sofa, in the corners of the room. No baby. I tore up the uncarpeted wood stairs, headed
for what I had been warned over and over was the most dangerous room in
the house—the bathroom. In case you didn't know, the disproportionately
large melon-heads of babies make them top heavy, so they can drown in a
bucket of water. Now, I can't imagine why someone would have a bucket
of water just sitting around their house waiting for babies to fall into. I
mean, what's the purpose? In case you are struck by a sudden urge to mop
the floors at midnight and don't want to wake people up by running the
sink? However, I did have something that resembled a bucket of water—a
toilet. Which didn't have a child lock on it, because when I had my allotted
twenty-three seconds to pee I needed the only toilet in the house to be easily
accessible, and besides, I was the only one in the house reliably using the
toilet on a regular basis. I raced up the stairs to the Toilet of Doom with Big
Pants following after. Of course, that was where we found the baby—sitting
in front of the open-lidded toilet looking quite pleased with himself. And
that was how we learned that Tiny Pants could crawl up the stairs.

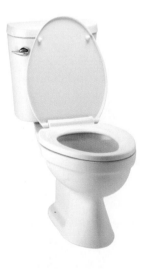

Dating as a Single Parent

1. Being a single mother means wearing cute, impractical shoes while lugging a toddler and baby to the store, because you never know when you'll meet someone.
2. Being a single mother means flirting with people that might be able to perform home repairs or change your tire.
3. Being a single mother means noticing whether every adult you come in contact with is wearing a wedding ring or not.
4. Being a single mother means thinking long and hard about who you allow to know where you live.
5. Being a single mother means realizing you don't need another husband, you need a nanny.

• • •

Before I left Daddy Pants, I poked around a little on dating websites. I did not write anyone, call anyone, or even open an account—I just wanted reassurance that if I left him, there would be dateable people out there. I figured I'd only be single for six months to a year. Not exactly how it worked out. You know how looking at houses online is a total roller coaster of hope? Everything is bright and shiny, and it never rains on Zillow. There are no bad smells on the internet. And everything is freaking perfect. People shopping is the same way.

• • •

I want to add a few cautionary words about dating as a single parent. Many of us returning to the dating scene are not up to date on internet safety. I was once chatting with a guy and he pulled up my previous home address online. I was terrified. I thought I was using an anonymous email address. I thought I was being safe. Luckily, nothing happened to me, but this is what I learned:

1. Most people have one good picture they like of themselves, so they use it as a profile pic across many sites. Don't do that. Someone can do an image search on Google and instantly find all the occurrences of that picture, like your Facebook account, or your company website.

2. Google the person before you meet them. It's not foolproof, but sites like dirtsearch.org can be helpful. Depending on the public records policy of the state you live in, you can also confirm their marital status ahead of time. It turns out that some divorces are more in the wishful-thinking stage than the actually-existing-in-real-life stage.

3. Tell someone the name of the person you are meeting for a first date and when you expect to return. Because my kids went to their father's house for three consecutive nights, I could have gone missing for days before anyone raised an alarm. Now, if you hate the idea of telling someone whom you are meeting, at least write down their name and contact info and leave it on your dining room table. It will give the police somewhere to start if you vanish off the face of the earth.

4. Drive yourself, or if you feel comfortable having them pick you up the first time, at least walk to a public place and meet them there so they don't know where you live. I know, we all say that we would never let someone we've never met pick us up, but sometimes after a month of talking to someone, you feel like you know them. You don't. There is nothing shameful about using Uber, Lyft, or old-fashioned taxis.

5. Google yourself. I was surprised to find that my work address and phone number were my top search result. Knowing what someone else can find out about you can help you decide how soon to share things like your last name.

• • •

Internet dating is really not more dangerous than meeting some dude at a bar. I mean, random people can still follow you home and kill you. I don't think any of us should live ruled by fear, but it's important to realize that the world can be a scary place, and I never wanted to put my kids in danger. The family safety rested on my shoulders alone, and seeing as I wasn't planning on moving any time soon, I kept people away from my house until I trusted them.

• • •

Once you find someone or a few someones to date, you may want to chitchat about them with your friends, like you did back in high school. I found that for these conversations, other single moms are your best bet. I expected judgy moms when I left Daddy Pants. I knew my decision was inexplicable to many mothers. Luckily, I didn't find nearly as many of them as I had anticipated. I think all married people have considered divorce on at least one occasion, so they didn't aim a lot of scornful glances my way—at least in public. I didn't particularly care what they said about me in their own living rooms—that was their right, as long as they were polite when they saw me.

What surprised me was that all the supportive married mom friends with whom I chitchatted over cookies suddenly fell silent if I mentioned the words "date" or, heaven forbid, "boyfriend." Eyes glazed over. Spines stiffened. Muffins fell out of mouths. Apparently, I was supposed to spend every waking moment atoning for my divorce by living in abstinence. I should have made a shrine to my children and sacrificed small body parts (my fingertips, or toes perhaps) when the children were at Daddy's house.

I get it. I've been divorced twice, so I don't exactly have a track record of making fine decisions to fall back on. When you readily admit to being twice divorced, married moms don't always think you should rush back into the dating life. To outsiders, my life probably looked rather like a train wreck. Life was slightly overwhelming, in the way that earthquakes, tornados, and children in diapers and armed with Sharpies are slightly overwhelming. And honestly, more children are abused or killed by boyfriends and stepfathers than by anyone else. I understand.

Still, I had standards about what I required in a man, and being good parental material was one of them. I know everyone says that, though, so I had a credibility issue.

• • •

One of the problems I have with society in general is that we tend to classify mothers as asexual beings with no needs besides the desire to nurture others. Stay-at-home moms judge women who go back to work full-time, because how could they leave their precious darlings just to feel fulfilled/pay all their bills in the same month/escape and get to talk to grown-ups? We also judge mothers who wear short skirts/tight jeans/whatever we can't fit into anymore because mothers are fucking holy. We can't hold in our heads the idea that women can be both loving/nurturing/devoted parents and also still retain a separate identity that includes wanting fun and sex and love and someone to hold them at night. And the loudest objectors to single mothers who date are the unhappily married women who feel trapped, at least in my experience. They need to believe that their decision to stay in a bad marriage is better than the alternative, and I was a prime example of the life they felt was out of their reach.

There's something else, though. Children look to their parents for relationship role models. They learn how to treat others based on how they see their parents treat each other. While devoting the rest of your life to your children and never dating sounds good in theory, it leaves a hole in their life when it comes to modeling adult relationships. I wanted my children to see how two adults that liked and respected each other interacted. And I never, ever wanted them to stay home from sleepovers or sports camps because they worried I'd be too lonely without them. Kids are amazing creatures, but it is not their job to be an adult's only companion. So I dated, and although I tried to keep my dating life separate from my Mama life, there was some crossover.

A few months after I became single and had moved into our new house (thanks, Mom!) I obtained a boyfriend. A truly nice and good person, as proven by the fact that although we liked each other very much, we just didn't have that magical love chemistry. Our relationship petered out after a few months. I can make good decisions, but I still require a certain amount of chaos for relationships to sparkle. Anyway, let's call this man Pasquale. I've never dated a Pasquale nor met one in real life, so it's safe. Besides, it's totally fun to say: *Pasquale.* I'd love to see someone in a porn/romance movie named Pasquale just for the bedroom audio. Pasquale had been divorced an entire ~~lifetime~~ year and so had already learned something about dating as a single parent. He had two girls, a few years older than my boys. Pasquale had already made the mistake of introducing his kids to someone who then broke up with him and it was far more traumatic for his kids than anticipated. (OK, that was a different Pasquale, but the point is still valid here.) Anyway, he had strong grown-up and completely rational opinions about not meeting children until we were "sure" about each other—although being divorced ourselves should be a clue that even sure things don't always work out.

However, I had very valid concerns about going through the effort of falling in love with someone just to discover they completely sucked with children. I had two stepmothers with my mom and four and a half stepmothers with my father, so I actually know quite a bit about the stepparent/child dynamic. My father liked to wait until the night before we made our summer pilgrimage to his house in Alaska to tell us that he and the most recent what's-her-name had gotten divorced. My brother and I fell asleep basking in visions of a summer with Just Dad, no evil stepmothers. It felt like Christmas Eve, but with an eleven-hour flight before we could receive our present.

Unfortunately, as soon as my father picked us up from the airport, he'd break the news that his new "lady friend" was waiting at his house and eager to meet us. *Fuck.* Then we spent the entire summer fighting the new what's-her-fuck for Dad's attention.

I felt it was important to test-drive Pasquale in the kid department before I did that whole *I can't live without you let's live together forever and ever* thing—when I could still back out. I had this amazing plan: I would have a housewarming party and invite a bunch of people over, one of whom was Pasquale. That way I could see how the kids reacted to him without them knowing that he was a date—Big Pants in particular, since Tiny Pants still only spoke in Cave Baby grunts and gestures.

I invited my best friend, Asterisk, her boyfriend, and her three children over. Pasquale showed up and we did not come within three feet of each other. We did not sit on the same sofa, which was tricky because I only had two chairs and one couch. I'm not sure that we even made eye contact once. Imagine my surprise when Daddy Pants texted, "I'd appreciate if you didn't bring your boyfriends around the children until you have been dating them for at least two years."

What the fuckity?

"Big Pants said that Mama had a party and her boyfriend was there."

Spies. They are everywhere.

• • •

Here is what I made for Pasquale the one and only time I cooked for him:

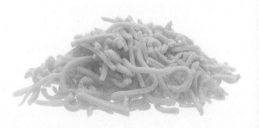

Mexican Lasagna
(It's actually called
Chicken Sonora or something like that.)

Ingredients

Chicken. Like a pound? Whatever a package is at the grocery store that seems to be a reasonable size and not too expensive. I buy chicken tenders (raw) because (A) they are cheaper and (B) half the cutting is done for you.

1 package of tortillas. You actually really only need half a package, but they come in handy to make wraps for lunch, so it is worth investing in a whole package. Besides, my store doesn't sell half-packages of tortillas.

1 package of taco seasoning

1 can chili (no beans)

2 bags of shredded cheese. You probably only need one, but cheese is love and you never want to run out of love so I always buy two. Officially it's probably supposed to be something like pepper jack or Mexican or whatever, but I use cheddar because I like cheddar.

1 can refried beans

1 jar medium picante sauce. You could obviously use hot or mild, but for some reason, my store seems to stock only medium.

Procedure

1. Cut up some chicken and boil it. Or fry it. I had always boiled it, but when I made it for Pasquale I thought I

(continued)

would fry it because it seemed more like cooking. What I didn't know, having never fried chicken before, is that it has to be DRY. I rinsed the chicken and threw it in the hot oil, which made a large popping whoosh and covered his kitchen cabinets with oil all the way to the ceiling. Just boil it, it's easier. Or buy the precooked chicken that comes in packages already diced. They stock them near the hot dogs.

2. Rip up tortillas. Layer in bottom of 9 x 11 pan, which I most likely should have told you to spray with cooking spray beforehand.

3. Layer on the chicken. Probably all of it. Shake taco seasoning on top in some approximation of even distribution.

4. Add a layer of that can of chili no beans. (After first opening the can, *duh*.)

5. Sprinkle liberally with cheese. Cheese is love, remember?

6. Add a layer of ripped-up tortillas again.

7. Next, spread the cold refried beans with a spatula or other such spreading device.

8. Add cheese.

9. If you did not yet run out of chicken and the pan is not full, add more chicken.

10. If you had some extra chicken, hopefully you thought to save an appropriate amount of taco seasoning to sprinkle on again.

11. Cheese. More cheese. Cheese forgives all cooking errors.

12. Bake in oven at 350 degrees (another thing I should have told you at the beginning of this, but I'm assuming you have cooked something before and knew to read through the recipe before you started. If not, no worries, just throw it in the cold oven, turn it to 350, and have a drink while it heats up. Doesn't have to be alcoholic. Milk is good, if you're not lactose intolerant. Or juice,

whatever. Of course, if you want an alcoholic drink, I recommend a margarita).

13. Turn on the oven light and look through the window.
When the cheese is melty, it is done. If you remembered
to preheat the oven, this is accomplished in something
like 10 minutes. If you are like me and completely forgot
to preheat until you got to this step, 20 minutes is your
magic number. Really, looking through the oven window
is your best bet.

ONLY MAMA

HOME | POSTS | ABOUT THIS BLOG | ABOUT ME

I Clean the Fridge and Ruminate About Marriage

I cleaned out the refrigerator today. I mean like I took everything out and washed the shelves kind of clean. If you know anything about me, you'd know this is not a common occurrence. It's not that I don't value having a clean refrigerator, it's just low on the priority list compared to, say, anything else in the world I could possibly be doing.

While I was cleaning, it occurred to me that cleaning the fridge is a fairly adequate metaphor for divorce.

OK, so you have this fridge, because you are an American and practically all Americans have refrigerators, and they are expensive, so you are pretty much stuck with the fridge you have. One day you notice it has a funny smell. Maybe, if you are like me, you stick your head in and look for the smell, and if the source of the stench of death is not readily apparent, you throw in a few boxes of baking soda, close the door, and hope for the best.

You wait. The smell has returned or, more likely, never left in the first place. You avoid going in the fridge. You make the children get things from the fridge for you so you don't have to open it. You spend a lot of time wishing you had kept up on fridge cleaning so you would not be in this position now. Perhaps you go to Smelly Fridge Therapy to try and work through your issues with the fridge. (Hey, it's not a perfect metaphor, work with me here.)

Eventually you have to face the fact that your fridge smells, and will continue to smell unless radical action is taken. So you empty the fridge and take stock of all the accumulated crap in there that you were previously unwilling to get rid of. It becomes apparent that most of what you have been storing is stuff that you don't need, don't want, or that used to be good but isn't anymore. Some of the items you throw out make you sad: there's the produce you bought and intended to eat but never got around to, the leftovers that are now a moldy memory of a nice dinner you once had. But you do it. You face your food baggage with courage and tenacity and a lot of Clorox bleach.

Once your fridge is empty, you clean the walls, the shelves, the little plastic door thingie that holds the butter. At this point, you very carefully take out each shelf and pay close attention to where it came from, and try to commit to memory the way the shelf slides into the latch thing so you can put it back together again. Somehow or another they never go back in the way they came out. Rebuilding your fridge is a whole lot harder than disassembling it. Sometimes you have to ask for help, like to figure out how the ice-maker drawer thing with the giant metal corkscrew in it goes back in. And sometimes you just have to figure it out on your own.

In the end, your fridge is clean, but all that work has made you aware of every little ding and dent and scratch in it that you never noticed when it was overflowing with moldy cheese and old pizza. If you are like me, you look at your fridge, and you are proud of the work you did, and even though it is a little bit dented and scratched and imperfect, it is more yours than when you started—you have examined and scrubbed and hand-dried it and you and the fridge have come through this experience together. And you both hope this time you'll do the preventative maintenance to never let the smell build up like that again.

You make a mental list of what you need to replace, and you close the door. Now you notice the outside of the fridge needs a little work. Maybe a new outfit and some highlights, but once the inside is in order, that seems almost fun. You scrub the door handles and wonder why on earth you didn't do this sooner, because you feel

(continued)

so much better when the outside looks nice. You look at all the preschool art that is curling up at the edges, and consider taking it down while no one is looking, but instead find some tape to affix it more firmly and attractively. After all, a fridge without finger paintings and crayon drawings is a cold, impersonal fridge, which you would never allow in your house.

So now you have a glowing, clean, empty fridge, which is patiently waiting for you to fill it up with fabulous, exotic new food, plus a lot of Diet Coke and those disgusting Go-GURT things your kids love but you aren't even sure count as food. You can fill it up with the same old leftovers and condiments, or you can leave it empty, only restocking what you need and truly want to keep.

. . . .

Posted by Lara L Monday, January 7, 2013 at 3:01 PM
Labels: Grown Up Time

Halloween and an Ill-Fated Facebook Romance

Big Pants was three years old and all he wanted was to be Barney for Halloween. I wasn't sure why this obsession was nestled in his heart but he was resolute. Only Barney. It wasn't that much to ask for really—the year before he got to pick anything he wanted to be. And I bought him costumes frequently—Buzz Lightyear, a monkey, a firefighter. Or I had, when I was married.

But my toddler didn't know that I was stringing together two part-time jobs so we could pay our bills and could continue to be mostly a stay-at-home mother, or that our cozy new house was subsidized by my parents, and although Daddy Pants did pay child support, I had to be careful, and purple dinosaur costumes were slightly beyond my grasp.

Tiny Pants, who had just learned to crawl, didn't have any opinions about costumes, or if he did, he wasn't making them known to me. Unlike when Big Pants was born and I had pored over baby costume catalogs, this time all I wanted was something that fit that I could afford.

I wanted to do this mothering thing right. It was all I had wanted to do since I was a child—I didn't have career goals, only this burning desire to have children. I didn't want to fail my son, particularly due to my decision to leave his father. I could sew simple things and we had access to many cardboard boxes. Unfortunately, a purple dinosaur was beyond my creative abilities. I tried to talk Big Pants into various other options, but he wouldn't budge. This was only a few months after I left Daddy Pants, and my child's world was all upside-down and I couldn't bear to crush his dreams. But I didn't have the forty bucks to spare, and I wasn't going to go into debt for Halloween.

· · ·

I called my favorite consignment store, conveniently located across the street from Big Pants's preschool, but sadly, they had no dinosaur costumes, purple or otherwise. In fact, they said that they had very few costumes left at all. After I dropped Big Pants at preschool, in a downtrodden dinosaur-less state of desperation I went to see what I could find before they ran out of everything in his size. Maybe I could find something almost as good. My mother always said that God looks out for fools and drunks, but apparently he also looks out for 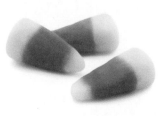 single mothers when his schedule allows, because smashed between two princess dresses I spotted a purple tail. No freaking way. Barney. Size 3T. Our universe was saved! They only had one costume left that would fit seven-month-old Tiny Pants—bizarrely, it was a fly costume with iridescent wings, but babies look adorable in anything, so I snatched it up.

· · ·

I did what many moms did on Halloween—posted a photo of myself and kids on Facebook. The boys were in their Halloween costumes—Big Pants's face was framed by the Barney headpiece, and Tiny Pants crawled around the floor in a teal fly costume with shimmery purple wings. I had accepted pretty much everyone who had friend requested me from high school—Facebook was still new and exciting to me. People commented on how cute the boys were in their costumes, and then I got a post from a random Pasquale saying how hot I was.

Random Pasquale sent you a message: "I'm trying to flirt with you, damn it!"

I was over the moon. I had had the biggest crush on this particular Pasquale for all of junior high. I had marched next to him in band—both of us playing snare drums, me enthusiastically but with inadequate skill, and him with the ease and precision of a natural musician. It is important to note that he never glanced my way once. I was too uncool with my big glasses, braces, and horrible fashion sense. I'd like to say I played coy, but within a few hours of receiving the message I called and teased him about what a jerk he had been to the little geeky girl. Within a few days we were talking on the phone for hours and texting constantly. I sent him an essay I had written—a sketch of how I had dreamed my life would be. He responded to the effect that he wanted to fit into my world. Within a week we had moved on to "I love you" and "Is this real?" And "I've never felt like this before."

Now, here's the thing. We have all heard stories of people who reconnected with old crushes on Facebook and eventually married them. That wasn't my experience. There is something visceral and magic about some people that makes you want to be around them every waking minute—this is what makes one person our best friend as much as it makes someone our crush—but it can't be faked, and it can't be seen online. It turns out, if you didn't have chemistry before—either love chemistry or friend chemistry—it is unlikely to have spontaneously evolved in the decades since you saw them last.

This man and I hadn't seen each other in fifteen years. We didn't know each other one iota, but what you do in these long-distance situations is spackle any gaps in your knowledge of them with your dream person. After three excruciatingly long weeks of texting and talking on the phone, what we had were two half-real, half-imaginary people who seemed to be soul mates but still were basically strangers. Everyone is perfect online—you never have a bad hair day, leave the toilet seat up, or bitch about toothpaste in the sink. If you're romantic and needy, it's the perfect way to build someone up into something they aren't, which is great until you meet them and all your hopes are smashed to bits.

We decided we *had* to see each other. It was Daddy Pants's turn to have the boys for Thanksgiving, so I made a plane reservation to go to California from Thursday at noon until Saturday at noon, so I wouldn't miss more work than was necessary. I sold my engagement ring to pay for the ticket, which may sound sad and wistful to someone else, but to me it was found money and I was happy to be parted from that cursed diamond. I wanted to be someone who flew across the country much more than I wanted to hold onto old memories.

From the moment I walked off the plane, I could tell that it was going to be a disaster. He was getting a parking ticket as I approached the vehicle, and was in a tizzy about it. I'm not the kind of person who sees any value in arguing with police officers, or in shouting "Have a Happy Thanskgiving!" sarcastically at said officers while gesturing with one's middle finger raised. I had woken at 3:00 a.m. to shower, shave my legs, straighten my hair, and do full-on makeup before boarding my plane at 5:30 a.m. West Coast Pasquale was wearing sweatpants and hadn't bothered to shave.

It became readily apparent that he didn't dig me at thirty-five years old any more than he dug me at age thirteen. He was still cute, but since we had never spoken back in high school, I didn't realize how completely incompatible we were. If we had run into each other at a local coffee shop, we would have had one of those, "hey, how are ya?" fifteen-minute conversations and moved on, but I had flown across the country and neither of us had any other plans for Thanksgiving, so we became actors in a reality show called "Let's Pretend We Really Like Each Other," which translated into eating a lot of fast food, watching a lot of movies, and taking naps. When it was time for me to return home he said, "Call me when you go home and we'll go from there." I called once I was back in Cleveland and he didn't answer or call back. I didn't yet know that "we'll go from there" was guy-speak for "I'll never talk to you again." (He was not the last person to use this exit line.)

In short, if you think you've discovered your soul mate on Facebook, and only mere happenstance kept you apart way back when, keep in mind that although it may be true love, it may just as likely be a near miss. You may discover that you feel about as much connection to them in real life as you do to an anonymous fish in a pet shop aquarium. Or you feel attracted to them and they look at you like you are the unpleasant fish/sad ferret waiting to be adopted. If you didn't have chemistry then, you probably don't have it now, either.

ONLY MAMA

HOME | POSTS | ABOUT THIS BLOG | ABOUT ME

Pawning Off My Work on My Four-Year-Old

I had no blog ideas today, so I decided to make Tiny Pants do my work for me. (I also got him to vacuum.) I don't keep a Mama journal of cute things he said, so I thought this might sort of serve as capturing a moment in his developmental history. Or something. Apparently, he wasn't much in the mood for being particularly witty and entertaining, either, but at least I can blame him if the blog post bombs.

Question: How tall is Mama?
Tiny Pants: Thirty-nine.

Question: Thirty-nine what?
Tiny Pants: Thirty-nine and a half.
(Well, now, that clears things up.)

Question: How much does Mama weigh?
Tiny Pants: Five pounds.
(not even close, but kinder than a lot of guesses he could have made)

Question: How old is Mama?
Tiny Pants: Thirty-nine.
(correct)

Question: What is Mama really good at?
Tiny Pants: Homework.

Question: What is Mama not so good at?
Tiny Pants: Playing catch. You get hit in the head with the ball a lot.

(continued)

Question: How are you and Mama the same?
Tiny Pants: Cuz we are in the same family.

Question: How are you and Mama different?
Tiny Pants: We aren't different. We are exactly the same.

Question: What is your favorite game to play with Mama?
Tiny Pants: I would say my favorite game to play with you is pig.

Question: How do you play pig?
Tiny Pants: You pretend to be a flying cow. You said I could say a made-up game.

Question: How tall are you?
Tiny Pants: One.

Question: How much do you weigh?
Tiny Pants: Zero.

Question: How old are you?
Tiny Pants: One.

Q: You're not one.
Tiny Pants: Yes I am. The ski mask is new so I am one.
(Ah, the youthful exuberance from new clothes. I know it well!)

Question: What are you really good at?
Tiny Pants: Looking at magazines to look for stuff to get for my birthday.

Question: What are you not so good at?
Tiny Pants: Catching or throwing or hitting a golf ball with a golf club.

Question: What's your favorite thing in the whole world?
Tiny Pants: You.

. . . .

Posted by Lara L Thursday, February 7, 2013 at 11:31 AM
Labels: Times I Got It Right or Just Got Lucky

I Encounter a Weird Married Mom

When Big Pants was in preschool, I had to go to these ~~stupid~~ adorable parties where all the moms pretend to care about talking to each other when really all we want to do is send our precious darlings somewhere long enough to take a nap. We also know that preschool is two years long and there's really no point in bonding with these people because when you get to real school there'll be a whole new bunch of moms there that you'll have to bond with because you'll be stuck with these new moms for the rest of your children's school years. OK, maybe all moms don't feel that way, but I certainly did. In my opinion, preschool moms were like practice moms and really, napping was more valuable. (Confession: one of the above-mentioned preschool moms sent her kids to the same school I did which made me rethink my judgment on preschool moms and also hope I was somewhat engaging at the blasted parties.)

Anyway, I had to go to this school party because you know, I love this kid I gave birth to and for some reason it was important to him. Actually, I would love him even if someone else gave birth to him because he is truly an outstanding child, and if I'm going to do all this work of parenting a child it doesn't matter much whether or not I actually gave birth to him. The truth is, I really did give birth to him in a long and painful experience and therefore I tend to refer to him that way, no offense to any adoptive parents. I digress.

This party was not for any particular holiday—because that would be politically incorrect—but instead was labeled something like the Spring

Cultural Banquet. I think they decided to do this because the class had started to make a dragon for Chinese New Year except it took them way longer to make the Chinese dragon than they intended, so in the end the party was nowhere close to actual Chinese New Year, and no one at the school knew of any other Chinese holidays to celebrate so they made it a cultural mashup. The kids proudly paraded their dragon throughout the room and then we ate food representing the holidays of the world, or something. I brought artichoke dip, because I always bring artichoke dip.

• • •

The party was in March or April, and it was cold, so I wore my orange velvet mock turtleneck and a long denim skirt, because long denim skirts are one step up from jeans and make it look like you are trying without actually having to iron anything. (I lost my iron for two years after I got divorced—it was in the cabinet with the cleaning supplies—somewhere I did not venture very often, apparently.)

At the party, some strange mom came up to me and said, "Can I pet you?" She immediately ran her hand up and down my arm while telling me how soft I was and how much she loved velvet. It was awkward and kind of creepy, because the only other time random strangers petted me was at a bar back in my twenties, and it turned out that the random strangers were on X. (I believe X has a hipper-sounding name now, but I'm out of that whole scene, and was actually never in that scene to begin with. Forgive me if I date myself by calling it X.) Anyway, if she was on X, she had no business being at a preschool cultural celebration. If she was not on X, she had no earthly reason to be petting a complete stranger's arm.

We exchanged some small talk and I said that I was a single mother. I had decided as soon as I got divorced that I would own my story and not shrink away or hide the fact that I was divorced. I figured the only way to meet other single moms was by letting them know I was in the club.

"Oh, you're a single mom? That's so interesting!" she purred, as she petted my sleeve.

"I have the funniest story," she continued. "I have this friend, and—Oh my God, this is hysterical! She and her husband both got sick *at the same time*. And it was the stomach flu, like coming out both ends! And they have two preschoolers. So all they could do was give each kid a box of cereal and turn on the TV. And they were sick for like twelve hours. When they finally managed to get out of the bathroom, their entire house was covered in cereal! Like the whole living room—the sofa, the floor, the chairs! Like it had snowed Cheerios! But what could they do? They got sick **at the same time**!" Creepy mom paused for me to laugh.

"Yeah, that's kind of what happens every time I get sick, because, you know, I'm a single mother," I said.

• • •

Here's my recipe for the above-mentioned artichoke dip, which looks like a lot of work, but isn't. Plus, I really like it, so if no one else does, I can eat it all. It also makes a fine stand-alone dinner when the kids are at their father's house.

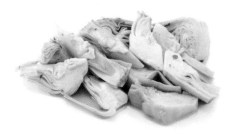

Artichoke Dip

Ingredients

1 can artichoke hearts in brine. You can buy them in oil, but when you pull them out of the can with your fingers, the hearts are slimy. I hate touching slimy things, and also meat on the bone, but the last part is irrelevant.

Parmesan cheese. The stuff you have in the back of your fridge is fine. Nothing special. You need something like ½ a cup if you have managed to not eat the entire can of artichoke hearts. If you only have ¼ cup of cheese left in the can, just use half the can of artichokes.

Mayo. I buy the squeeze kind because I hate washing dishes and the squeeze kind means you don't dirty a spoon getting it out of the container. You can also use reduced-fat mayo with no negative consequences.

Procedure

1. Open can, drain artichoke hearts. If you dump the can of drained hearts onto the cutting board, you'll be surprised by how much juice didn't drain from the can, and if you ignored my advice and bought hearts in oil, this makes a slimy mess, which I warned you about. Sometimes that's all there is available on the shelf, though. I choose to use my fingers to extract the hearts and eat some of them as I go. If you do use the finger-extraction method, use caution around the sharp edge of the can.

2. Chop up the hearts. They really don't have to be that finely chopped. I aim for chunks no bigger than a square centimeter, but if there are a few bigger chunks it's fine, because I for one really love when I find a bigger chunk in artichoke dip.

3. Put chopped-up artichoke hearts in bowl. Not a huge bowl, but not a kid's bowl. Like a soup bowl or slightly-larger-than-regular bowl. (This may seem like a stupid inclusion but only if you've gotten sleep. If you're a single mother, a good night's sleep is like a unicorn sighting. People who don't sleep appreciate things that are spelled out clearly.)

4. Pour approximately an equal amount of cheese as you have artichoke hearts into the bowl. I don't measure because I often eat half the hearts while cooking.

5. Squeeze the mayo on top of the other two ingredients. Again, aim for roughly the same amount of mayo as you have cheese. The ratio is 1:1:1. This might not be Betty Crocker's ratio in that easy recipe book, but Betty also added onion (which I'm against) and assumes that I keep my measuring cups in my kitchen, instead of the living room where the baby was always playing with them.

6. Mix it up with a fork. Use the fork to squish up the artichokes a bit.

7. Cook in microwave for a few minutes until it bubbles. You may expect more precision, but microwaves vary greatly. Remember, watching through the window is truly your best bet, because then you don't have to remember cook times.

8. Serve with tortilla chips. If you don't have any, you can substitute with pita, chunks of bread, pretzels, Ritz crackers, Wheat Thins, Triscuits, or Dinosaur Chicken Nuggets. You can therefore bring dip to a party and assume that someone else will have provided the necessary scooping device. Not that I recommend that strategy, but I can't say I haven't done it.

Nannies versus Husbands

When I first went back to work, my best friend, Asterisk, watched the boys for the one and a half days a week that I needed childcare, but soon she got a day job and I had to find someone new. I only worked outside of the home part-time, but most places required full-time attendance. Plus, Big Pants went to Montessori school half-days, and I didn't want to pull him out to put him in an all-day center. We had no family in town, but the kids still had to eat, so I was going to have to find someone who was more flexible—preferably another mother.

It's scary to think about hiring a complete stranger to watch your kids, and since I had only lived in Cleveland for a few years, I didn't have a large group of friends to ask for recommendations. I did what I did when I was looking for a boyfriend—I went online. I found my beloved nanny on a website that functioned like a dating site for parents and independent childcare providers. The website ran background checks, provided references, and clearly listed hourly rates. Surprisingly, women who could bring their own children were often willing to work for far less than the teenagers I occasionally hired. Nannies were not just for the well-to-do.

A normal person would have interviewed a nanny at their own house, seeing as that is where the person would be watching your kids. They might need to know how to find your house, where to park, and where you keep the toilet paper. Oh, and they might meet your kids first. For some reason, I felt I would learn more about her if I saw her house and met her child, who was in between Big Pants and Tiny Pants in age. (Her kid was sleeping during the interview, so that was a fail.) Plus, I was leery of giving people I met on the internet my address—even potential nannies—without meeting them first.

The first thing I noticed was that she had lots and lots of toys nicely put away in her living room. I didn't trust people who had children but no visible toys. The fact that she was capable of keeping them neat and I so obviously wasn't seemed like proof that she knew important mothering secrets that I didn't. I also noticed that she had a nose piercing. I didn't personally have a nose piercing but I did have bright unnatural scarlet streaks in my hair. I have always liked people who refused to restrict themselves to society's box of what mothers should and shouldn't look like. It made her more interesting.

I don't think I asked unusually brilliant questions. I remember some discussion about religion (she's Hindu, I'm Unitarian) and about why neither of us planned to homeschool but admired people who did. I liked her and felt comfortable around her from the very beginning. But what made me know for sure, 100 percent, no take backs, that she was the right person to watch my kids was her cat.

• • •

Nanny had a cat with a crumpled ear—more specifically, a mean cat with a crumpled ear. Anyone that could go to the pound and decide the crumpled-ear cat was the one they couldn't live without was the person for me. I did call her references, and I ran a background check. I am not entirely stupid. Basically, though, I was won over by the cat.

Nanny was amazing. She parented my kids the way I would have. For example, on the first day she took them to a playground, but she selected a fenced-in playground so they couldn't escape. Not knowing my kids, this was wise. Tiny Pants, just two at the time, came home with a red mark on his eye from walking around with a stick. (The white part of his eye, not the lid, for your visual reference.)

We had some sort of conversation like this:

"I just wanted to let you know that Tiny Pants has a red mark on his eye because he was walking around the playground with a stick," Nanny said.

"OK, well, I would totally let him walk around with a stick. Explore nature and all that," I replied.

Some might think this was a bad start, but it wasn't. I do want my kids to climb trees and experience the world with their hands. If they are going to get injured, I'd rather it be the kind of injury they'd get under my supervision—as opposed to something like a chemical burn from washing the floor on their bare knees. A cleaning-induced injury is highly unlikely to occur on my watch. Poking eyeballs with a stick is.

Nanny became like family, and her son was like a cousin to the Pants brothers. She saw me on the days I could barely pull it together to go to work, and she'd do nice things like the dishes without being asked. Once she cleaned my microwave as a surprise. My kids love her to pieces and didn't even cry when she came over.

Beloved Nanny moved away, so I found a college girl. She did not own a cat with any deformations, but she seemed nice. She was willing to drive all over hell's half acre to pick up the kids from various schools. That relationship ended when I caught her rummaging through my dresser drawers.

Luckily, Nanny moved back to town (thank God), and we had a few years of blissful co-parenting one or two days a week. She was the person I discussed parenting concerns with, like how to con the boys into eating healthy food and whether or not it was reasonable to expect them to clean up after themselves. Sometimes I'd come home and she'd have that same crazy-eyed look I get, but she'd always smile. She never threw things at my head after a long day, even though sometimes I'm sure she'd have liked to. Once I went out to an evening hockey game with my friend Herman and left her with the kids, and Tiny Pants got a bloody nose, then her son puked on Tiny's bed. She still came back. I don't think I could have been that strong.

Now husbands? Haven't had so much luck there. Here's a secret I'll share: I suck at compromise. I have really zero interest in it.

Daddy Pants and I had a few major parenting disagreements. One was on letting the baby cry, and one was on how to diaper the baby. I had one way to solve all parenting debates: you don't bitch, and I will do all the work. I told Daddy Pants, "Here's my plan. I will do every single night feeding/comforting. You don't argue with my parenting choices." He agreed. Who wouldn't? But that attitude—the *my way is the only way* attitude—is not fine co-parenting. Apparently it's not so great as a relationship strategy, either. I don't regret that decision—I just realize that if you are going to refuse to compromise, a nanny is a better option than a husband.

If you ask the nanny to wash the baby, they wash the baby. If the nanny disagrees with your parenting style or if you are mean to the nanny, the nanny leaves. This is sad, but there is no nanny divorce court you have to go through. And because you know that the nanny can evaporate at any moment, a smart mother is exceedingly grateful to her nanny and loves her and tries to always keep her nanny gruntled so she will come back the next day. I couldn't have gotten through the early years without her.

Actual Letter to Nanny on Her First Day on the Job

April 11, 2009

Dear Nanny,

All the diapering materials are in the box by the TV in the living room—wipes, diapers, plastic bags for stinky ones. In the boys' room I also have diapers and wipes so you don't have to drag stuff between floors.

> Warning: Bogie eats poopy diapers! He begs when you change Tiny Pants. I do not let him eat them, and if the dog says otherwise he is lying!

BIG PANTS

Fully dresses himself—I let him pick his own outfits, but occasionally have to veto shorts in winter, etc.

Bathroom—completely independent, even with overalls, but for some reason announces that he has to go.

"Mommy, I have to go potty!"

"OK, go."

"OK, Mommy!"

That's all the involvement he needs, other than a reminder to flush and wash hands.

Big Pants can be trusted to listen and not get into stuff he shouldn't, not run off, etc. Big Pants talks nonstop, but he really wants to be obedient. It is completely OK to tell Big Pants it's time for quiet time when Tiny Pants naps. I generally give him the choice of some independent activities (watch TV, play with Leapster, do a craft). I don't ask for quiet time every day, but it's perfectly acceptable.

DISCIPLINE

I'm a big fan of threats. With Big Pants, it's generally enough to say "We won't do ____ if you do ____." I never hit or spank. I do employ the time-out occasionally, more with Tiny Pants than the Big One. We don't have a particular "naughty spot." Anywhere will do. I use the rule of one minute in time-out per year the child has been alive.

I *try* and have the boys clean up before we leave the house. The goal is to get the toys off the floor so Bogie won't eat them.

I am not horribly big on rules, but I am very big on manners. Even Tiny knows "Peeze" and "Dank oo." Tiny Pants will give you something and tell you "Dank oo," because he thinks "thank you" goes with getting or giving something. He's so cute.

FOOD

In spite of what they say, they do not get cookies for breakfast!

Dry cereal in a bowl is my standby. They snack a lot, which is OK. Do not feel like you ever have to cook, but if you like to, I generally have muffin mix, pancake mix, etc. Big Pants LOVES to ask for something and then not eat it.

Tiny Pants will not take soy milk in a cup for me, I don't know why. He only gets soy milk at nap/bedtime. At some point I need to stop that but don't really know how. He loves water though. Neither like juice, though Tiny likes to squeeze the juice box all over the table, so watch out!

Lunch tomorrow will be mac 'n' cheese for Big Pants and plain noodles for Tiny. If they object, they can have peanut butter and jelly. I like to give them a choice of two things if I can. I feel like that gives them a degree of control over their life and leads to less arguing just to assert themselves. It might be completely untrue, but sounds good, right?

TINY PANTS

Tiny Pants is a holy terror. He can open the cabinets, microwave, children's Tylenol, etc. He loves to open purses and scatter stuff throughout the house. He is a kid who loves funny noises, so if he steps on you and you go ouch, he'll do it again, and again. Tiny Pants has to apologize to whomever he hits. He is a sweet kid, really, just at *that* age.

Tiny Pants's naptime—bottle of half soy/half water. Clean diaper and in the crib with him. He'll put himself to sleep—generally around noon, sometimes before lunch.

BOGIE

Bogie eats toys. Bogie eats everything.

Bogie will run away. He's fast. You have to hold his collar until the leash is fully engaged or he will take off.

Bogie will growl if he is sat on, jumped on, etc. I feel this is fair.

One thing I hate about Bogie is that he will take food out of Tiny Pants's hand. You can gate him in the kitchen anytime, particularly when they are eating.

Bogie is allowed on the couch, but he knows "off, move," etc. I have little patience for being sat on by the dog all day.

I am fine with you taking them places, just please send me a text of what you're up to, or where you are going. I am also fine if you stay at home all day. There is a potty seat and step stool in the bathroom closet. Big Pants doesn't really use the potty seat anymore. Tiny Pants doesn't really use the potty. Feel free to potty train him if you like. (That was a joke. Probably.)

Grocery Shopping

When you are a single parent, everyone you know will give you dating tips, and one of them is to always look cute at the grocery store because you never know who you are going to meet. This is eerily similar to the advice I was given when I was previously single and not yet a mother. Apparently, the grocery store is the hip place to pick up people.

At eighteen, I used to drive past the nearest grocery store to go to the Official Singles Grocery Store. I never met a person there, not once—not even when I snuck a kitten in under my jacket, which I can honestly say I don't recommend because they have claws and they squirm and are really hard to keep from dropping when you are holding them inside your coat. Generally, cashiers are pretty excited when you sneak kittens into the grocery store (which I have actually done on more than one occasion) but they aren't much of a dude-magnet. No one has ever asked me to leave for kitten-smuggling, but no one asked me for a date, either.

Even though we all know that no one ever meets anyone else in the grocery store, enough people will advise you to always look cute at the grocery store that you'll feel guilty shopping in sweats and will instead wear cute jeans and boots. The only thing this will accomplish is that you may slide all over the place in the parking lot while pushing a cart containing two small people through the snow, but you'll do it guilt-free and can report to your mother that you always look cute in public and therefore it is not your fault that you have not yet found anyone new.

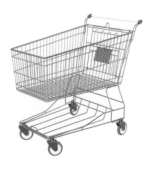

The benefit of shared parenting is that you can go to the grocery store when the kids are at Daddy's. You can shop like a grown-up. You can buy wine or beer or cigars if you choose (if grocery stores sell cigars, which I'm not sure that they do, seeing as I don't smoke cigars) without people looking at you like you are a terrible parent.

Here's a secret: nearly every single parent I knew smoked. Even the nonsmokers had a secret pack of cigarettes tucked away in a cabinet or on top of the fridge to sneak when children weren't around. I'm not saying they smoked regularly or in front of their kids, or anything like that. For some reason, single parenting turned us into a bunch of teenagers. I had not smoked in five years when I became a single mother, but I was mooching cigarettes within a month. Pretty soon I was buying my own. I'm not saying that smoking is a good life strategy, or that I did it for very long. I'm just saying life is stressful, sneaking bad things somehow makes you feel young, and coughing allowed us to punish ourselves for the permanent single-parent guilt we all carried. I did try very hard never to buy cigarettes in front of the children, not because toddlers had any idea what they were, thank God (and also thank God toddlers didn't know what tampons were, either), but because all the other grown-ups in the store did, and they were really good at judgy looks, and I was very bad at deflecting them.

You know what else you get judgy looks for? Buying condoms. Which, if I saw my younger self buying condoms while accompanied by two kids in diapers I'd be so happy I'd buy them for me myself. Which doesn't make sense, because it would still be my money, but it would be future/older me's money, not younger/poorer me's money. Now, you might think people would say, "Look at that woman with two kids and no wedding ring—thank God she's using birth control and being wise about STDs!" No. Mothers are never allowed to sin in the checkout line.

The problem is that going to the grocery store is a complete and utter waste of precious Grown-Up Time. Besides, when the kids are at Daddy's you can eat any freaking thing you want for dinner, including cereal, so keeping proper groceries in the house was not absolutely necessary unless the children were home. Plus, most divorced parents are on the Divorce Diet.

The Divorce Diet is a real thing. It has to do with being too stressed out/exhausted to eat properly and is a real weight loss/gain strategy that seems to be unavoidable. The time crunch and stress level of single parenting leads many of us to under- or overeat, or both on alternating days. We have guilt. We have angry texts and lawyers and, if you live in Ohio, a mandated shared-parenting class. Although food was extremely high on my children's list of priorities, it often felt unnecessary for me personally. My Facebook status frequently read, "Lara doesn't need food. Food is for the weak." It wasn't that I was purposefully starving myself—I also posted, "Lara doesn't need sleep—sleep is for the weak," quite often. It was more a marveling about how little I actually needed to get by. I had always been a sleeper and a snacker. I was now a get-lost-while-driving-to-work-because-you-are-overtired-er, and a subsist-on-microwaveable-dinners-and-caffeine-er. I got down to below my high school weight in a few months without even trying.

Although stress accounted for a lot of it, some of my weight loss was due to the fact that kids only need air and three graham crackers to survive, and the graham crackers are mainly used for entertainment purposes. So when I made dinner for kids who ate one dinosaur chicken nugget apiece, I tended to put less on my own plate, because I didn't even remember what a grown-up-size portion looks like. But there's a downside to rapid weight loss—excessive skin. From outside my clothing, I looked twenty-eight-ish. Beneath my clothing, I looked seventy. In reality, I was thirty-five. I liked being thirty-five, but I wanted to look thirty-five without my clothing. For the first time, I become a fan of indirect lighting. You know what else indirect lighting is good for? Hiding dust on bookcases, televisions, and other horizontal surfaces. When I finally put weight back on, my skin filled in again, or filled in enough that I was willing to turn the lights on, but then all the dust became visible.

• • •

One lesson my friend Asterisk taught me was that Tostitos Creamy Spinach Dip and chips are a completely appropriate grown-up meal. This relieved me of any and all guilt over my own nutrition. It has spinach and some sort of creamy substance that must have calcium and maybe even protein in it. Therefore, healthy. Queso dip? Also fine—it has cheese and some pieces of something that looks like a pepper and are therefore vegetables and that also equals healthy dining.

Due to my lack of culinary skills, I tried to eat out, get takeout, or eat leftovers for at least two out of the three kid-free dinners shared parenting afforded me. I also tried to eat at non-kid-friendly establishments, or at least places my kids refused to go. Some people's kids eat grown-up food. No judgment, but I think they may be aliens. Mine did not eat any chicken that was not in the shape of a dinosaur nor mac and cheese that wasn't fluorescent orange. Apparently, these two staples are in short supply at most dining establishments, so I had many choices when the boys were at Daddy's. Sometimes I couldn't bring myself to leave the house once I got home from work. On these nights, if by chance I didn't have an adequate supply of dip and chips, I found myself eating ramen noodles or Easy Mac or some other non-grown-up substance, which then meant I had to drag the kids to the grocery store the next day because I ate the only four things they were willing to consume that week. Of course, I would have to wear cute boots just in case I met someone.

One thing I was a huge fan of buying was egg whites that came in a carton, because they were easy to pour and lasted for freaking ever. I could stock up once a month and never worry about them going bad, and then I never had to crack eggs. Cracking eggs isn't a terrible amount of work, but I have an unusually high fear of salmonella, so cracking eggs requires excessive handwashing and counter spraying with Formula 409, and when you have a baby and toddler on the loose in the living room, that takes an extraordinarily long amount of time. Plus, egg whites have fewer calories than regular eggs, so I use the calories I saved for chocolate consumption. In the yolk calories versus chocolate calories debate, chocolate always wins in my house. But plain egg whites look like the kind of breakfast that is only appropriate if you are wallowing in self-pity. I generally eat brussels sprouts or kale when I'm wallowing in self-pity. Breakfast is supposed to be a reward for being awake, so I became an expert in the breakfast concoction.

My Ultimate Egg White Breakfast

(Also Known as Mama's Breakfast Concoction)

First, you need a carton of egg whites. They can be Egg Beaters, store brand, whatever. Note: Egg Beaters are yellow and therefore slightly less creepy than the clear ones that magically turn white while cooking.

1. Take whatever nonmetal bowl you'll eat out of, spray with a little bit of cooking spray if you have it. If you don't, you'll live—you'll just have to scrub the bowl harder. For some reason I always make my eggs in a Tupperware container instead of a real bowl, even though I have real bowls available.

2. Pour egg whites from the carton into the bowl. How much depends on how hungry you are and how much you have left from yesterday. There's an egg equivalency chart on the carton.

3. Add a spoonful or two of leftover dip from your grown-up "dinner" the night before, or any other random snack item in your fridge. Choices include:

    (a) Salsa
    (b) Tostitos spinach dip
    (c) Ranch dressing
    (d) Sliced pepperoni
    (e) Blueberries (they are actually really amazing in eggs but turn the whites a funny color)
    (f) Meatloaf. I know it sounds weird, but it's actually delicious.

(continued)

4. Add cheese, because cheese is love.
5. Pop in the microwave for not too long. Try 45 seconds, then stir. I have been betrayed multiple times by egg-white concoctions that looked done on the outside but were still runny below the surface. So trust me on this, stir, put back in for at least 20 more seconds, but do not forget to remove the metal spoon! Note: you will not blow up the microwave if you forget to remove the spoon unless you have maybe gone upstairs to take a shower or something. In general, the sparks and explosive noises will quickly alert you to the omission of this very important step. Again, looking through the window saves lives.

The Big Fat Truth About Cleaning and Being Single

I try to keep my blog fun and upbeat, but the truth is there are a lot of sucky parts of being a single parent. Of great sucktitude is having to be the one to do everything.

I may have bitched once or twice about my ex not doing "enough," but he did contribute; he worked, I stayed home. I cleaned the house, he mowed and shoveled. We once lived for ten months in an apartment building during which time I never managed to learn where the dumpster was, so therefore never had to take out the trash.

Here is today's sample: pick up kids, make dinner for kids, stop making dinner to plunge toilet, continue making dinner after sanitizing hands thoroughly, wash dishes, play with kids, shovel snow, do homework, bathe kids, play with kids, make kid do homework, put kids to bed. Cleaning doesn't happen very often, yet I feel guilty about the state of my house. If I get a free hour I nap, I don't clean.

I decided not to do any more laundry until all of the existing laundry is folded and put away. We are now nearly naked.

Oh, and I backed into a telephone pole this week, with Tiny Pants in the car. Thankfully he was not hurt, nor traumatized. I was slightly traumatized, I have to admit. I swear, that pole came out of nowhere. The fact that I had no idea it was there disturbed me

(continued)

greatly, so I did the only sensible thing—I blamed the car. It really does have crappy visibility, but in general, inanimate objects are not at fault. Well, that's what they tell me.

I tend to get really pissed off about the state of my workload, but I also know I am far better off than most single mothers. I don't work three jobs to make ends meet. I get to actually spend time with the kids when I have them. I also don't have an asshole boyfriend who lives with us and makes my kids' life a living hell. I also don't have a nice, sweet live-in boyfriend they have to compete with and therefore act out and induce feelings of maternal guilt. There is much to be thankful for, really, but self-pity is so much more fun than gratitude!

———————————

Here's my poor-me list:

I have to do all the shopping, cleaning, cooking, home repair, mowing, shoveling, laundry, oh I can't go on. It's too much to list. I can't bear it.

But here's some truth:

Husbands, in my experience, seem to have different cleaning schedules than I do. For example, they want me to clean the most on days I have absolutely no interest in cleaning. If I don't want to clean, I don't, and there's no one to criticize. I can let the dishes sit for a week, ignore mountains of laundry, and take the kids to McDonald's PlayPlace instead of dealing with it, and no one can stop me.

Husbands also tend to have a different view on where the dirty laundry goes. I vote laundry basket, not floor. I used to have four laundry baskets in the bedroom in strategically located places to make laundry throwing easier, but it still didn't work. Daddy Pants looked at me one day and explained that it wasn't his fault; his laundry feared the baskets, and he didn't want to traumatize it.

I don't have the resentment of expecting someone else to do something, nor can I angrily blame someone else when I can't find something. I may get frustrated with the chaos, but I know it is my fault/responsibility. This actually makes me happier in the day-to-day moments.

There's also no yelling at kids because they will make someone unhappy with their mess. No frantic cleaning before Daddy comes home. No turning down the television and tiptoeing around a boyfriend.

If we choose to have a blow-up boat in the living room for a week, no one complains. Or a potty chair in the living room. ("Mama, I made a poo-poo, and Dog disappeared it.")

It is *my* mess! I shall revel in it! And if I choose to go eat cookies in bed and leave the mess there till morning, I *can* and I *will*. And what do I hear when I do so? Pretty birds singing in my head. No yelling. No evil looks.

Pretty soon the boys will start cleaning up (I hope). They love to shovel, and soon they will be big enough to mow. I will get to do all the gleeful yelling at the children to clean up, something I have been looking forward to for years. I will get to skip gleefully around the living room barking out instructions. I may even make myself a drill sergeant hat and buy a whistle. And I won't have to share my whistle.

. . . .

Posted by Lara L Friday, January 25, 2013 at 9:02 AM
Labels: Not My Finer Moments

Housekeeping

1. Being a single mother means relaxing your cleanliness standards. A lot.
2. Being a single mother means missing your kids like crazy when your ex has them, only to want to give them away ten minutes after you get them back.
3. Being a single mother means accepting sleep deprivation as a natural state.
4. Being a single mother means letting your kids eat off the living-room floor.
5. Being a single mother means sometimes not doing dishes for a week.
6. Being a single mother means doing a mountain of dishes before you get your first cup of coffee.

Some people clean when they are upset. I am not one of them. I think my life would probably be improved if I at least occasionally cleaned when upset, but unfortunately I'm too nice of a person for that. You see, my laundry is scared of the dark. If I put it in drawers or closets it'll have nightmares and I just can't bring myself to sink to that level of meanness.

Here's the problem with getting kids to clean: they suck at it. And I have to admit that I don't "see" mess the way other people do. In my opinion, "clean" equates to clear space. Meaning, if my table has several carefully stacked piles on the table and 75 percent of it is clear, it is clean. (If there's no coagulated ketchup, obviously. I'm not a monster.) The side table overflowing with stuff? I don't look at it. It is not the focal point of the room, therefore it doesn't matter. When I was a kid, I had to clean the dining room table. I carefully made a pile of all the scattered papers, then cleaned the table with Pledge. Same with the piano bench and piano—straighten the crap, clean around it. Slide the pile to wipe underneath it. Ignore the side table overflowing with crap, because it had Important Things Never to be Touched by Children on it, like bills and stamps and rolls of undeveloped film. When my stepmother came to visit she took one look at my house and said, "I'm afraid we failed you by never teaching you to clean properly." I should have said, "Damn straight you did, now hire me a cleaning lady!" Of course, I didn't say anything of the sort, because I was too busy being insulted. Sadly, it was a missed opportunity.

When the kids were under the ages of six and eight, I sporadically tried to get them to pick up their toys. This involved me standing over them and giving step-by-step instructions: take that truck, put it in the cabinet. No, don't play with it. Now pick up all the markers. All the markers. Stop drawing on your face. Put. The. Markers. In. The. Box. This approach made cleaning an all-day project, and not only did the house not get clean, but no one was happy. It devolved into, "torture children, frustrate Mama, and wind up with a still-filthy house!" So basically I just ignored the mess until the kids went to Daddy's, then I spent the rest of the day cleaning. For a few days, my house was clean, except that side table in the dining room, because who the hell looks at side tables in dining rooms? Serial killers, that's who. People looking for easy escape routes after they have murdered my family. (The side table in question is directly under a high window, which I guess is relevant if I want you to understand my "serial killer escape route" reference.)

I even mopped sometimes. Unfortunately, no one ever came over when my house was clean, because when the kids went to Daddy's I worked all day and went out to dinner if I could swing it and spent as little time as possible in my living room. When the kids were at Daddy's, the sight of one left-behind toddler-sized mitten shredded me into tiny pieces.

Within five minutes of arriving back at my house, the children needed to reassure themselves that all their toys still loved them and hadn't been traumatized by their imprisonment in the toy cabinet, and so it was truly vital that they take every toy out and give them air to resuscitate them. Tiny Pants would look at me like, "Wow. That was close. If I had been gone another day, my one-legged Batman action figure would have gone into a coma from oxygen deprivation. Thank God I came home when I did because obviously

Mama does not care at all if Batman suffocates and dies in the dark." And then he'd fill his diaper and run laughing around the table. I'd have to chase him and strip off his diaper and forget that I moved the wipes when I tidied up so I'd hold the baby down with one arm (on a blanket on the floor) while I tried to reach the wipes with the other arm or possibly my left foot and then I'd notice the dog had found the cloth diaper and cleaned it out for me. And then I wasn't sure if I should be grossed out (obviously) or grateful because now the dirty diaper was still disgusting but also less stinky.

Of course, while all this was happening, Big Pants pulled all the books off the shelf and then lost interest in them and was demanding a snack, because my kids ate every 12.5 minutes on average. Seeing as I had to go into the kitchen to put the cloth diaper in the pail and wash my hands, I might as well get him a bowl of Goldfish Crackers so he could eat three of them and scatter the rest artfully around the living room, because they really are pretty and we should all enjoy them. Besides, then he would have effectively given his baby brother a snack, too (thanks, Big Pants!), because babies are perfectly happy eating Goldfish off the carpeting.

Before I had kids, I had a friend who was a single mother of a four-year-old boy. I went to her house after work one day, and she put her kid in front of the TV and dumped his McDonald's Happy Meal on the floor in front of him, fries and all. I thought this was not only lazy but bizarre and unsanitary. I didn't know then that it was an economy of motion, because if she put the fries on the table he'd just carry them into the living room anyway and drop them all on the floor. At least with her technique, the fries were all in one place. I never poured French fries on the carpet intentionally, but I did pour them on the coffee table. Yes, without a plate, even. So far, the kids have lived.

One thing I did not allow, if I could help it, was sharing of food with the dog. I did not care for the idea of my precious offspring eating dog-slobbered fries. However, our dog was quick and I was sleep deprived and so it happened. The dog would take a piece of pizza out of my kid's hands and chew on it, and before I could stop him, the boy in question would grab it back and take another bite. I would make a gargled *yaaarg* sound and take the pizza out of the boy's hand and try not to puke and give him a fresh piece of pizza.

Cleaning Tips for Slackers
(Best Done in the Order Provided)

1. Lock the children in the closet until you are finished cleaning, or their eighteenth birthday, whichever comes last. Tell them it's a fort. Kids love forts. (My lawyer insists that I need to remind readers that I am being funny and don't actually advocate locking your kids in the closet. I told my lawyer that if the reader doesn't understand my sense of humor we have a lot more problems than just this chapter.)
2. Don't bother picking up the toys on the floor, just vacuum around them. When company appears, act surprised at the mess your children made while you were taking a shower. (This works best only if you have remembered to let the children out of the closet before guests arrive.)
3. Wet down hair to make shower excuse plausible.
4. If it smells clean it is clean. I worked in a gift shop with a twentysome-thing man who chanted this over and over as he sprayed Windex in the air instead of wiping down the shelves with it. Also, this gives you the excuse that the overpowering smell of cleaning detergent gave you an allergy attack, so therefore you can only entertain in the backyard.
5. Take a laundry basket no more than half-filled with laundry and per-form a one-arm sweep to clear everything off your table into the basket. Hide basket in the basement.
6. Hide dirty dishes in the oven. (In truth, I have not resorted to this, but enough people have recommended it that I must include it.)

7. Scatter important-looking books around to provide justifiable reason for your mess. (Try to keep impressive titles like *Business Law* or *Calculus* around just for this purpose.)

8. Make expansive arm movements and talk nonstop when guests arrive to distract them.

9. Only invite date-type people over after dark and light candles.

10. Become friends with someone whose child is a clean-freak. They will organize your children's toys for you when you send them all upstairs to play. (Thanks, Asterisk.)

Note: The results are mixed on whether having a dog is beneficial or not in terms of home-cleanliness. I did not get my dog back (my parents borrowed him for a few years) until a year after I had started single parenting, so I have experienced life both with and without a dog-helper.

Positives:

1. Dog eats any and all crumbs/spills/food dropped on the floor or his head.

2. Dog empties potty chair.

3. Dog assists in dirty diaper cleaning, as noted above.

Negatives:

1. Dog also eats food on the dining room table and knocks over milk frequently when doing so.

2. Dog sheds everywhere.

3. Dog eats crayons and produces multicolored poops in the yard, which are easily spotted by company who may or may not appreciate rainbow excrement.

Conclusion:

Deciding to purchase a dog should not be based solely on their cleaning contributions.

My First Single-Mama Mother's Day

I wasn't looking forward to my first Mother's Day as a single mama. Since my parents lived out of town, there would be no Mother's Day brunch with my own mother. Big Pants was three, and I was still carrying Tiny Pants around in a car seat carrier. I looked at everyone's "Happy Mother's Day" posts on Facebook and just felt hollow.

I knew my kids loved me, but I also knew there was no one to help them make me a card or anything. Heck, Tiny Pants would probably chew on a card, anyway. I felt selfish for caring about a stupid Hallmark holiday, but I did. Mother's Day just emphasized how alone I was while everyone else was with their families.

Big Pants attended preschool, and they were putting on a Mother's Day program called "Muffins with Mom," or something like that. I figured it would probably be long and dull and just accentuate how different and alone I felt as a single mama. But when Mrs. S. came to my car window at pick-up and asked me directly if I was planning on attending, I didn't know how to say no. I explained that I worked at a church, so we would be late, but I promised to show up. I was dreading it.

Church had been the only place I went where I could relax and talk to people, confident that someone would keep an eye on all the toddlers running around the room and make sure none of them escaped into the parking lot. Once I started working there, though, church became somewhere I had to be upbeat and cheerful. I could no longer lean on people the same way. By taking the job, I lost the only support system I had. I wore a skirt to church in honor of Mother's Day, but I performed my job by rote that morning—smiling, talking, shaking hands, but feeling like I was an empty husk of a person. All I wanted to do was take a nap and wait for the day to be over. After church, we went to the preschool's Mother's Day program, and I tried to make small talk, but I felt like an alien—a different species of mother. They looked suspiciously well-rested and well-ironed. These moms all had husbands at home who probably helped their children pick daisies in the backyard and make toast, or at least let them shower on their own. I was glad when they served the muffins so I had an excuse not to kibitz any longer.

After we ate, the teacher turned on a CD player. As "You Are My Sunshine" started to play, Big Pants handed me his gifts: a fake flower arrangement in a small vase that he had assembled himself and a macaroni necklace. He sang along in his baby-talk voice that still couldn't say the letter R very well. I started to cry small and secretly, but luckily we were outside and I was wearing sunglasses. He was too young to understand happy tears. I wore my macaroni necklace proudly, and protected it from Tiny Pants's sticky fingers. It was everything I ever wanted. When I got home, I put my noodle necklace in my jewelry box, and the vase of flowers in my cabinet along with my most cherished objects. After that, I didn't stress about Mother's Day so much. There was always a teacher ready to force my children to make something to bring home to me, and it was a great excuse for us to all go out for breakfast together. I paid and drove, of course, because they were still too short to see over the steering wheel and not skilled enough at anything to land a decent job, but I also learned that Bob Evans will give mothers free carnations on Mother's Day, and I am a fan of free flowers.

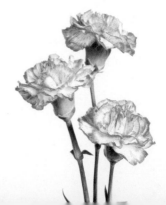

Moms Gone Wild

I was speaking to the newly separated father of one of Tiny Pants's friends the other day. He was baffled by his soon-to-be-ex-wife's behavior. He seemed to think she was acting kind of crazy. I told him that I went kind of crazy after my separation, too—at least from Daddy Pants's perspective.

I think society likes to put women into boxes, and once we enter the box labeled "mother" we are no longer seen as people. We are expected to give up everything for our children and family. As young women we are offered only two boxes: virgin and whore, and as mothers, we are born-again-virgins by default. While it might sound nice to be viewed as pure and holy, it's a lonely existence. Divorce allows many of us to redefine ourselves, and for many of us, this newfound freedom is exhilarating—which might make us come across as a little crazy to our ex-husbands. It's okay to go a little wild—even necessary, I think. But here's some advice on going wild based on my own missteps.

Many of my married mom friends say that they are happy that they came of age before the internet, and *yay, them,* but those of us reentering the dating world in our thirties are not so lucky. Did you know people can screen-grab still pictures of you off of Skype? Not, of course, that I ever did anything on Skype that seemed inappropriate at the time, but taken out of context I had plenty of reasons for late-night anxiety. Notice I said, "Seemed inappropriate at the time." That legally gives me plenty of wiggle room.

. . .

Someone once told me that you stop emotionally maturing when you are in a relationship, and while I think that is probably pure bullshit, it is plausible that your dating maturity remains the same as when you last were single, before you met your future-ex-husband. So, if you met when you were twenty and divorced at thirty, your dating IQ is likely still that of a twenty-year-old. While of course you were a very mature twenty-year-old, you have to realize that all the newly single men out there are also stuck at the dating IQ of their premarital ages. The idea that we are all mature adults now makes me laugh and laugh at my gullible younger self. We weren't. I wasn't. I thought I was, but no no no no.

Something I didn't know beforehand was that everyone lies on the internet. Before I left my (then future) second-ex-husband I went on a blind playdate with a single mother. I had met her in an online writer's group, and she was solo-parenting two boys almost exactly the same ages as mine. I needed to know how this whole single-mama thing worked IRL. I had seen pictures of her online, so I figured she wouldn't be hard to spot. I mean, how many platinum-blond high-school-skinny five-foot-tall mothers could there be?

Zero, it turns out. She was not blond. Not skinny. Not recognizable in any way, shape, or form from the pictures I had seen online. She laughed about it. "Not what you were expecting, am I? All my pictures are of me. I just know how to angle the camera."

I can honestly say that I never photoshopped a picture of myself or posted an obviously out-of-date picture, but I only posted my best snaps, where the light blurred my wrinkles. If my arm looked fat, I'd crop it out. And it turned out that men played these tricks as often as women. I submit the following quotations as evidence, all told to me by one man or another:

"Yeah, the picture may be a few years old, but I basically look the same."

"I *am* athletic. Not all athletes are the same size."

"If I posted a real pic, no one would date me."

It's not PC to say we have physical standards in dating. We are supposed to see the person, not the packaging when it comes to race, weight, height, and so on. This is all true when it comes to friendship, but the difference between compound words and single words like *boyfriend* versus *boy space friend* is attraction. Attraction has a physical component that can't be helped. Sure, people can become more alluring as you get to know them. I have been told that I'm not a head-turner but rather my looks grow on you, like algae. I'm not saying that dating someone outside your attraction range can't lead to true love and physical chemistry, but we all have deal breakers. Insurmountable obstacles we can't overcome no matter how fantastically charming the potential mate is. Like earlobes.

• • •

I have dated short men, tall men, skinny men, and chubby men. I have dated men of all different religions and professions, but I have never dated a man with attached earlobes. I just can't do it. I realize that people have absolutely no control over how their ears attach to their heads. The rational part of my brain understands that earlobes are not linked to intelligence, personality, or anger-management issues. The rational side, however, is a pushover when it comes to the sexual-attraction side of my brain. Earlobes aren't important, people tell me. I have a weird obsession, my mother says. It's not that I sit up nights admiring photo galleries of detached earlobes or anything, but ears are the first thing I notice on men, and if their earlobes are attached, I'm out. Interestingly, I have no idea if my girlfriends even have attached earlobes, including the ones I have kissed. This is strictly a male issue in my world (although I did snipe at my SigO that he should have known his marriage wouldn't work out because his ex-wife had attached earlobes, but I was just being catty).

The first man I kissed after Daddy Pants did actually have attached earlobes, but to the best of my recollection, he was the only male person with attached earlobes I have ever kissed. I had foolishly never zoomed in on his online pics because I had forgotten how detrimental earlobes could be to my level of attraction. I'll even admit that it was a fine kiss, maybe even one of the top-ten kisses of my life, but that was the end of it. There are some things you can't change about yourself no matter how stupid you know they are, and no matter how artfully a man hides his earlobes in his dating profile picture, the truth will come out the instant we meet and then it'll be a colossal waste of time, hope, and a child-free evening.

Remember that Moms Gone Wild thing I teased with at the beginning of the chapter? I'm getting there. First of all, it is totally normal to want to reclaim yourself as a sexual and beautiful woman. Particularly for mothers, as we are inundated with messages that mothers must be holy and pure and completely focused on their husbands and children. There are posts about what we can and can't wear after we have children, which have absolutely nothing to do with how well we can pull it off, and is only about the idea that mothers shouldn't still be women. I call bullshit.

• • •

When I was pregnant with my first child I realized that my window for being an exotic dancer had closed. I had never been an exotic dancer, and never really wanted to be an exotic dancer before, but when I was pregnant suddenly it seemed like I had missed out on a tremendous opportunity. Hormones are weird, and gaining fifty pounds in six months is weird, and realizing that you'll be responsible for another human being for freaking ever is weirdest of all. Mourning my loss of stripping opportunities was actually less weird, if you think about it in that context. I didn't really want to shake my moneymaker(s) on stage (I'm all tits and no ass). The feeling that I no longer would have the option to be outrageous, in-your-face sexual was horribly depressing, even if I had not previously thought it was something I wanted to do. I had given up my freedom in marriage and my body in pregnancy. I wished I had been more outrageous while I still had the chance.

But guess what? Divorce meant I could be outrageous again! I could do all those crazy things I never got to do when they were age appropriate! I didn't actually use the opportunity to become a stripper, because in the end it still wasn't any more "me" at thirty-five than it had been at twenty-five. I did however kiss girls at bars just to shock people. I dirty danced and flashed my bra to my best friend Asterisk and felt very risqué. It was fun and I don't regret any of it and I hope to God it wasn't caught on film. I also had a professional Facebook page for work and used a different name for my real Facebook, because employers look at shit like that. Unfortunately, I didn't realize that one of my Facebook friends was really Daddy Pants. Lesson: As safe as you think you are being on the internet, try not to get caught on film.

Free Tips for Moms Considering Going Wild

1. If you want to go wild by kissing a girl, that's fine. Don't go wild by kissing lesbians. They take girl kisses seriously, and when you wake up the next day you'll discover that you have seventeen text messages and also that you are a douche.

2. Do not go up to strange women and grab their boobs. I was wise enough to know that this was not liberation, but I have witnessed drunk women squeezing the Charmin of complete strangers. Even if you think of yourself as a mom going wild, it's still assault.

3. Men who say they don't mind if their wives kiss girls generally mean they don't mind only if they themselves are present. Some of them mind quite a lot if you kiss their wife when they are not present, but that's a different story altogether.

4. If your version of going wild involves karaoke or crazy dancing and you also are prone to anxiety, it is best to do it where no one knows your name and can't tag you on social media. I always use an assumed name when I forget I can't sing and sign up for karaoke—generally George, but sometimes Michael or Paul. I like to keep the DJ off-kilter.

5. The best thing I ever did for my self-esteem was to have some alluring pictures taken by a professional photographer. I was dating a man who I really liked but who was just keeping me as a fallback in case he couldn't find anyone better. Seeing photos of myself that were fun, flirty, and— I'll say it—gorgeous helped me lose interest in being anyone's second

choice. They were worth a hundred selfies. If someone leaks them on the internet, at least I am proud of them. You don't have to spend a lot of money—even having a good friend take some pictures for you is worth doing. If you go that route, take a lot of pictures in several outfits. If you are as critical as I am, fifty pictures = one or two useable shots. Seriously, we don't pay for film anymore, there's no reason not to take a heap of photos. As the camera clicks, don't just hold the same pose. Move your head subtly, drop your chin, or raise it. Look down, then away. You also don't have to show them to anybody else—they can be just for yourself. My sister and I shared pictures with each other when we were both single and needed an ego boost, and I'm sure we weren't the only ones.

6. If you choose to embrace your sexuality by going to a strip club with a bunch of girlfriends, it's best to call ahead. Some clubs require women to be accompanied by a man to gain entrance. It has something to do with wives dragging husbands home, I think. Remember that dancers don't work for free and don't want to be groped, no matter your gender. They aren't there to make risqué new friends—they are there to work. Even if they add you to their Facebook friends list, realize any time they spend sitting and chatting is time they aren't making money, and they pay to go to work. Show your feminism by tipping well.

7. Many cities have pole-dancing classes or other classes inspired by the exotic arts. These are definitely worth taking if you want to celebrate your sexuality and keep your clothes on. There are two downsides:

    (a) Poles can leave bruises and friction burns, and

    (b) you pay them; they don't pay you.

    I took something called aerial lyra, which is basically performing some pretty poses in a hoop suspended from the ceiling perpendicular to the ground. The instructor told me to grab the hoop—which was over my head—and pull myself up and into it. I grabbed the bottom of that steel hula-hoop thing, looked at my pitiful biceps, and thought that there was no way in hell this was going to work. Since there was no ladder and I didn't want to be the only person too weak to get into the damn thing, I jumped and pulled and kicked my feet and I managed to pull my body up. I learned to balance in the hoop holding on with just one hand, and then to point my toes and do graceful things with my legs. I felt strong and beautiful and even a little brave. The backs of my knees and insides of my thighs were covered with bruises, and I was proud as hell of them. It is still one of the best things I have ever done on a Wednesday night. Pole was discouraging for me, because I have the coordination and balance of a puppy, and never managed to manage even the simplest of maneuvers.

8. If you prefer to release your wild side through comedy clubs, go online and sign up to win tickets. Many places develop a list of people they call when the shows are not selling well. This gives you the opportunity to invite someone on a date, or bring several friends and look like a big shot. If you are the person who never has much money for frivolous things, being able to treat your friends on occasion is a treat.

Part of going wild is eating like a teenager, except that your taste buds have matured and maybe your sense of style has as well. Homemade tortilla chips made me feel much more accomplished and grown-up, but I was still basically eating chips for dinner. Plus, they go well with leftover dip of all kinds, so if you have no food in the house but do have some leftover tortillas, you can make something resembling dinner.

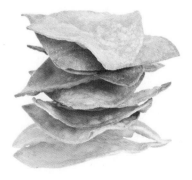

Homemade Gourmet-ish Tortilla Chips

I had these at a pool bar (swimming, not billiard) in Key West back when I was in my late twenties, and figured out how to make them myself. They are very good for impressing new friends and/or dates when you are just serving dip for dinner, especially if one chip gets an air bubble inside and swells up.

Ingredients
Canola oil, aka regular unfancy cooking oil. I do not know what a canola is.
Flour tortillas (corn would probably work, too, though I haven't tried it)
Clean scissors
Salt

Procedure
1. Heat oil in pan over some source of flame (not a microwave). Make the oil like ¼–½ inch deep.
2. While oil is heating, cut tortillas into strips with scissors. Long strips look more impressive than triangles.
3. Lay tortilla strips in oil. Overturning ruins them, so you have to wait a few minutes, then lift one corner and look to see if the strip is getting brownish and crispy. When it is, flip over and cook another minute or two. Really, just keep peeking. What else can you do with a minute or two? It's not enough time to wash dishes. You're in the kitchen anyway. Timers are for sissies.
4. Drain on a paper-towel-covered plate. Oil is now the enemy. Blot the top. Oil = soggy chips.
5. Salt liberally. Really, you can't have too much salt, because half of it slides off.

ONLY MAMA

HOME | POSTS | ABOUT THIS BLOG | ABOUT ME

I Swear, Children, I Never Flashed my Boobs at Fantasy Fest

I had the amazing fortune to attend three Fantasy Fests when I lived in Key West way back when I was young and child-free. Over the years we had a few lamentable mishaps (like when someone slipped X to a visiting houseguest, causing her to throw up for hours) but mostly it was fun in that Big Fun way you like to look back on and immortalize after you have children and can't really have that kind of grown-up fun anymore.

For those who are unaware, Fantasy Fest is a weeklong festival in Key West, attended by approximately eighty thousand people, many clad only in body paint and the scent of yesterday's beer. It's about cheap plastic beads in the same large way that Mardi Gras is. The goal is to get so many beads that you get a neck ache or at least a really sweaty collarbone from wearing them all night. Many women flashed their money-makers to get beads, but I did not.

I figured it wasn't really a thing locals did, because, unlike the tourists, I would have to see some of these people again, like at work or in the grocery store. I had a friend who flashed at Fantasy Fest, and she was confronted the next day by a homeless man who raised his shirt when he saw her and said, "I saw your boobies last night!"

I also knew that I was going to be a mother someday, and I didn't think that was the kind of behavior I wanted someone to catch on film and potentially haunt me with. Like many of my decisions, anxiety kept me in check.

(continued)

Also, you could not flash and still get a ton of plastic beads, so why bother? If they were throwing strings of rubies or pearls that would be another thing entirely.

In the divorce, I fought Daddy Pants for and won our joint Fantasy Fest bead collection, which we had toted around in a box in the half a decade after we left Key West. We moved seven times, and each time we carefully packed the beads up and brought them along. I let my ex win the fight over the kitchen broom and steam cleaner, but those beads were mine.

The beads have since become property of the boys and live in a tangled heap in their bedroom. Occasionally, generally when a girl comes over, they are brought out for dress-up or pirate treasure or what have you.

I found their ride-on ponies decorated in beads the other day, and I nostalgically untangled a few more strands for Spot and Butterscotch (the ponies) to wear. And then it hit me: someday these kids'll learn about flashing tits for beads at Fantasy Fest, Mardi Gras, or some other bead-greed parade, and they'll remember their mother's ginormous stash of beads.

It doesn't matter that I kept my shirt on—they'll never believe me. Heck, I don't think any of my friends now will believe me. I have evidence of a crime I never committed already stashed in the memory banks of my kids.

Essentially, I should have flashed everyone after all. Although, looking back, I don't regret not flashing. It would have been out of character for me in those days. And I still have boobs, old boobs, granted, but they are still attached to my body. If I really want to flash someone, I still can. Those kids aren't around every minute. My grown-up-fun days are not entirely behind me if I don't want them to be. I am not dead yet.

. . . .

Posted by Lara L Thursday, February 6, 2014 at 10:44 AM
Labels: Grown Up Time, Not My Finer Moments, Single Parenting, Times I'm Just Weird

On Naps

When I was in high school, sleeping was my favorite hobby, and I pursued it with passion. I tried to nap every day. My mother was kind enough to let sleeping teenagers lie, and I rarely ventured downstairs before noon on Saturdays. As an adult, I remained devoted to my sleep habit, and insisted on always getting at least eight to ten hours of sleep a night, supplemented with naps on the weekend. Then I had children.

Big Pants hated sleep from the day we took him home from the hospital. I nursed him every two hours for twenty months. Then I got pregnant for a second time, and it's fair to say that I didn't sleep again for five years. As a single mother, at first we all slept in my bed. Big Pants could only sleep burrowed into my side, his arm across my belly and tiny fingers tucked under my back. Tiny Pants preferred to sleep at the foot of the bed (he liked his sleep undisturbed) but would occasionally crawl to the top of the bed and drape himself over my head in a snuggly baby hat fashion. Eventually, I got them both into their own beds, but there were frequent night wakings and, after I stopped nursing, polite demands of "more baba please" long after dark.

Several of my friends managed to nap while their children were home, but I had never been able to do it. I just couldn't relax enough to actually sleep while my ~~demon-spawn~~ beloved children were jumping up and down on my back as I lay on the couch, the TV blaring Barney or Elmo. Besides, I had been horrified when a friend confessed that she awoke one afternoon to find her toddler in the backyard wearing pajamas and wielding a light saber in the snow. Every night that the children were home, I was awakened every few hours by one of them. You see, they belonged to the Don't Let

Mama Sleep Union, and by contract they were obligated to ensure that I never slept through the night. I'm certain that they conferred each evening as to who had which shift, so that between the two of them I was never asleep for very long and yet they both emerged fully rested each morning. When the children were at their father's house (and a normal person would catch up on sleep) I went on dates or out with girlfriends and had to wake early for work, so sleep didn't happen much then, either. However, I learned that four to six hours of uninterrupted sleep felt as good as eight hours of broken sleep. I thought that I was doing well, and that it was just a coincidence that I spaced out often and had a habit of missing my exits whenever I drove. (The benefit of missing my exit constantly was that I learned many alternate routes to and from work in a very short amount of time.)

• • •

A year after moving in to our tiny, happy single-mama house, I turned thirty-six. Big Pants was almost four, and Tiny Pants was only eighteen months old. I made myself a cake to share with the kids because it was my birthday and I was going to enjoy all the cake I wanted guilt-free. For some reason, instead of making it in an 8 x 10 pan like normal, I decided to fancy it up and made two round eight-inch cakes stacked on top of each other with a layer of frosting in the middle. This provided me with added festiveness as neither my first-ex-husband nor Daddy Pants had ever made me a stacked cake before, and it provided an extra layer of frosting, and I really needed an extra layer of frosting that year. Do you know those plastic cake-holder hatbox-looking things? I didn't have one, so I took my largest pot and placed it carefully over the leftover cake as a lid, and prided myself on my resourcefulness. Yeah, it was kind of heavy, but it worked and was free. My boyfriend came over after the children were asleep and we stayed up far, far too late talking on the porch. Like two in the morning late, not like ten thirty-five late. It was my birthday, and it seemed like a good idea at the time.

However, when Tiny Pants woke up for the day at five thirty the next morning, it no longer felt like such a great plan. There was not enough coffee in the world to make it through the day. We made breakfast and played Thomas trains and I changed diapers, then at about noon I lay facedown on the couch while my children enjoyed some quality children's programming. Big Pants promptly sat down on my back to improve his view of the television, and Tiny Pants stood at his play-table-thing and banged away at the attached squeaky buttons and twisty knobs. Somehow, I actually fell asleep.

"Mama, can we have cake?" Big Pants asked, his voice cloudy and far off. I made some sort of affirmative *hmphmm* noise and kept on sleeping. About an hour later, he woke me again, "Mama, I think the baby is eating your earring."

I dragged one eyelid open and saw that Tiny Pants did in fact have the end of one dangly earring hanging out of his mouth. I quickly grabbed it out of his drool-puss before he decided to swallow. I sat up and looked around.

It was as if a cake bomb had exploded in the living room. Big Pants had gone into the kitchen and somehow managed to lift the cake with its giant pot-cake-lid off the stove (which was above his head) and carried it into the living room. He carefully placed it on the coffee table where he and his brother decimated the entire thing. There were crumbs all over the carpet and the walls were covered with frosting fingerprints. Tiny Pants was licking frosting off the coffee table and Big Pants was on the floor, stuffing handfuls of cake into his mouth. All I could think was that nap was totally worth it.

The Mama Bus Always Leaves on Time

I hate to be late like my dog hates rain. Actually, I hate to be late as much as my old cat, Phantom, hated rain. Phantom was a stray my first-ex-husband brought home from the hospital where he worked—the cat was living behind the dumpster, and when the first snow of the season fell, my first-ex-husband rescued him, even though he didn't particularly like cats and even though we already had three, which my mother always told me was a few too many. First-ex-husband named dumpster kitty after the Phantom of the Opera, because he was a black "tuxedo" cat with a white mask over half his face. Because Phantom had been a stray, he didn't behave exactly like the rest of our cats. First of all, he beefed up to twenty-one pounds in a matter of months. Self-defense, I figured, in case of a(nother) famine. The other cats brought home mice and left them on the doorstep, because obviously I was too big and clumsy to hunt for myself. Phantom brought his kills inside because it was a safe place to eat them. I once walked into the kitchen and right there on my linoleum floor I found the cat chewing on the bottom half of a squirrel. And another time, while I was unloading groceries from the car, he dragged an entire five-pound hunk of raw roast beef to the basement and gnawed off a significant portion before I discovered him. (I washed it with dish soap and cut off the masticated edges, but still, no one would touch it when I served it for dinner that night. Cat spit is hard to purge from your mind.)

Besides his food issues, Phantom hated rain. Whenever we had the slightest precipitation, that cat would come running down the street, meowing his head off like he was being murderized. I called it Post-Traumatic Rain Disorder. You could hear him a block away. So as much as that cat hated rain, that's how much I hate being late.

I recognize that I would be less wigged out (and therefore my kids would be less wigged out) if I could allow for the occasional possibility of being late. Like, maybe the world won't end if we aren't early to everything. What am I saying? Just typing those words is giving me anxiety.

Anyway, we were invited to a birthday party at a new friend's house. I wasn't entirely sure where it was, and I know how much I hate when we have a party and it's time to start and no one is freaking there yet. Suffice to say, I felt it was important to leave on time. Except I couldn't find my boots—the ones I was wearing twenty minutes previously when I took out the trash. The black motorcycle boots, bought on sale at Target, were the only boots that fit over my favorite fluffy socks, and no way was I going to change my fluffy socks because:

A. It was cold,
B. They were my favorite mismatched stripe combination, and
C. Running upstairs to change my socks would make us late.

So the boys were standing by the door of our tiny one-thousand-square-foot house with their coats all buttoned up, and I was lifting up the sofa and digging under piles of toys (yes, this would have been easier if my house was ever actually clean) trying to find my boots. In an effort to speed up the process, I enlisted my tiny, perfect, angel children to help look in the kitchen, under the dining room table, and any other place that they could think of to find my boots. No joy. I gave up and stuffed my fuzzy-socked feet into too-tight other boots because again, I wasn't going to delay leaving even more to find the appropriate sock/boot combination the first time we were invited to someone's house who was probably watching the clock anxiously waiting for us to arrive.

We left. I took deep breaths. We drove to the party, which turned out to be only

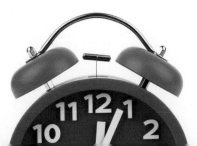

six minutes away (thank God). As we stood at the new friend's front door, I looked down at my two children for the first time. Big Pants was wearing sweatpants and boots and was relatively clean. Tiny Pants was also wearing pants (not pajamas like he normally did) but his feet looked kind of large and duck-like. On his feet were my motorcycle boots. The ones he helped me look for. The ones that nearly made us late, because I couldn't spare five seconds to look at his feet before we left the house. And now the door was opening and I had to explain to a mother that I had never met why my child had women's size-eight boots on his five-year-old feet. Luckily, she had three children and understood these things, or at least that's what she told me.

Single Parenting Turns You into a Teenager

When was the last time you made out in a car? If you are a single parent, it might have been last Friday. If you go home, you have to pay the babysitter and send her/him home. If the babysitter leaves and the kids wake up, there'll be no more kissing for you, and you really are in the mood for some kissing. And if you are at home and in the mood for some kissing, an alarm will sound in your children's bedroom and they'll come racing down the stairs to prevent this from happening at all costs.

You know what else you get as a single mama? Best friend sleepover parties, with a pile of sleeping children in one room and moms taking turns sneaking out or making phone calls or watching not-safe-for-children movies. Borrowing cute clothes and eating Fritos that you hide from the children. Sending my best friend upstairs when the children would not go to sleep and I worried I might break their precious eardrums if I had to tell them one more time to get back into bed. Dyeing each other's hair once the kids were finally asleep or at least quiet.

It was my girlfriends who saved me when I locked myself out of the house, or when my minivan broke down at the side of I-90 with the kids in the car. My childcare provider was my most significant other, the person I talked to about developmental milestones and how to get the kids to eat food that wasn't shaped like a random animal. My single-mama years were a championing of friendship that was never quite the same once boyfriends evolved into significant others.

I also got opportunities to do weird things high school me would have loved to do, but never was asked to do, like getting cast as a zombie in a college movie. Which sounded like a great idea until I found out that I had to be on set at eleven o'clock at night for hair and makeup because they could only use the mini-mart after it closed. Luckily, Asterisk approved of my zombie venture, and her kids were at their daddy's house. She slept on my couch and distracted my kids when I ran in at 6:30 a.m. to shower so my sweet adorable children would not be scarred for life from seeing their mother in full zombie makeup and clothing splattered with fake blood. After that, I swore I would never do another college movie, but when they asked again, I said yes, and got to be an Iraqi woman who returned from the dead to stalk a US Army soldier with PTSD. Unfortunately, it was never picked up by Sundance or anywhere else the director submitted it to, but it did win a couple of awards at the local film festival. I got all dressed up and drove across town for the film fest, which it turned out was only attended by six people plus the cast and a middle-aged bald lawyer who really wanted to buy me a drink. By then I had learned that it was far easier to refuse a drink than deal with the consequences.

• • •

I also made the unfortunate mistake (more than once) of trying to sing karaoke with a group of girlfriends who knew how to sing. I did not. Actually, I did know how to sing. I spent my teen years in various choruses—one of which I had to audition to join. So technically, I did know *how* to sing. What I did not know how to do was find the notes by myself. I was very good at singing quietly while standing next to someone who was singing all the right notes very loudly. On my own, however, I sounded like a sick cat or a dying cow, and the sad thing is that I know it. The first time I sang karaoke I was part of a foursome where the two peo-ple who knew all the notes held the microphones and Asterisk and I stood behind them un-mic'ed but very enthusiastic. Unfortunately, friends and wine insisted that I really did have the skill to sing my shower song, "Killing in the Name" by Rage Against the Machine. This was going to be my solo karaoke debut. I knew all

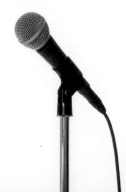

the words. It was a screamy song, so I didn't have to worry about hitting all the notes. I was ready.

I took the stage. The music started. I stood there looking at the words rapidly scrolling across the monitor and was unable to open my mouth. I realized the best way out of this predicament was probably to throw up or run off the stage, and if something didn't happen soon, fate was going to choose for me. Luckily, some random dude jumped up on the stage, grabbed me too hard around my waist, and sang along with me, loudly and not on key, but who cared? He saved me from public humiliation and I never did karaoke on my own again.

• • •

In honor of sleepover parties, zombie movies, and bad karaoke I give you:

Actually Healthy-ish Microwave Popcorn AKA Desperation Popcorn

My father visited me when Big Pants was five and Tiny Pants was three. I called home from work and asked him to pick up some popcorn, because everyone in the house liked it, and it required only one large bowl everyone could eat out of, and I did not have a dishwasher. Imagine my dismay when I returned home and instead of the lovely blue-and-white Pop Secret box, or the equally lovely red-and-white Orville Redenbacher box, or even the store-brand box of any color whatsoever, I found a jar of old-fashioned popcorn on my counter.

"Dad, I don't own an air popper," I said in what was probably not my sweetest, most grateful voice ever.

"Oh. Well, we could buy one?" Dad responded.

"No, it's fine, I'll pick up some microwave popcorn later," I answered, in what was most likely a very patient and loving voice, because I was a very patient and loving person, even if I had just got home from work and discovered that I had no popcorn. I stuffed the completely useless jar into my cabinet, because what else was I going to do with it? I couldn't throw it away—it was food, after all—and it would probably be good for filling beanbags or something.

Well, one day I wasn't feeling well and the kids were hungry, and no freaking way was I going to leave the house, so I took that jar of popcorn and poured some in a brown paper bag and threw it in the microwave as an experiment, because the air popper we had as a kid just swirled the kernels in hot air, and how was that different from a microwave with a built-in rotating plate? Not much, it turns out. It worked perfectly, plus there was no oil or hydrogenated stuff to feel guilty about. Nanny commended me for being so health-conscious. I managed not to laugh until she went home.

Ingredients

Jar of popcorn kernels like you bought when you were a kid and people used air poppers to make popcorn because microwaves weren't invented yet. Air poppers were a vast improvement over the stove-top method we had previously employed, and so popcorn became something we ate frequently.

Brown paper bag like we used to take our lunches in to school in the years after lunchboxes became uncool but before reusable scuba-material lunch sacks were invented.

Microwave. Because staring at popcorn kernels in a paper bag on the counter is unproductive.

Procedure

1. Pour ¼–½ cup of popcorn kernels into paper bag. Roll up end tightly. I suppose you could even tape the end closed if you were the kind of person who had both tape and brown paper bags in the house at the same time. (Clearly, I was not.)

2. Place in microwave (long side down, in case it matters) and turn on for a few minutes. As with all popcorn, you have to stay and listen for the pops to slow down because burned popcorn stinks up the whole house and also turns the insides of microwaves a weird yellow color that is very hard to remove. Plus, no one will eat burned popcorn except the dog and he's too fat already.

Kitchen Lies

When I was a child, my father fed us Chef-boy-oh-boy ravioli—the kind that comes in a can and permanently stains your cheeks orange. (It also permanently stains a shih tzu's fur orange, but that's another story.) He cooked it a very special way, so that some of the ravioli were warm, and some were hot, and some were kind of cold. He said that was the surprise of ravioli— you never knew what temperature it would be when you bit into it. I was in love with the magic of half-cooked ravioli, and when I went back to my mom's house, I asked if she could make it that way, too. I honestly did not think my mother was up to the task of the sometimes-hot-sometimes-warm surprise ravioli, but she knew exactly how to make it, also. I figured Dad must have taught her back when they were still married. It wasn't until I was in high school that I learned that most people (like my boyfriend at the time) cooked ravioli to an unsurprising even temperature. They also don't always make it from a can. I was bitterly disappointed on both accounts.

• • •

When Big Pants and Tiny Pants were young, they refused to eat just about anything that wasn't a carbohydrate. They'd snack out on crackers, cereal, toast, and cookies (the four food groups of toddlers), but if it had any nutritional value at all, they would act like I was trying to poison them. When Big Pants was a baby, he ate only jarred baby food, and he only ate sweet potatoes, carrots, green beans, peas, and something yellowish-orange called chicken noodle, which had neither chicken nor noodles in any recognizable form. Five items. I was hyper-worried about food allergies, so anytime I fed him something new, I would watch him all night for signs of fussiness. I also sucked at force-feeding him. I nursed him, so I considered food more of a novelty plaything than serious nutrition. Of course, when he graduated to real food, he refused to eat anything besides the four carb groups, and I entirely blamed myself and swore that the next time, I would do better. When Tiny Pants was a baby, I never fed him any premade baby food. I just gave him soft things I was eating, like bananas or avocado, and little mushed-up bits of things off my plate. I let him chew on a pork chop like a little toothless puppy. I was going to raise a good eater, and I did, until he turned three and inevitably joined the carb union with his brother.

One day, Tiny Pants announced that he wanted ham. I actually had ham in my refrigerator at that very moment! Okay, it was Canadian bacon, but technically, Canadian bacon is ham in my book. I could provide a protein source with the minimal amount of effort and expenditure!

"I don't like Mama Ham," he cried once he saw it on the plate. "I only like Daddy Ham!" What the fuck was "Daddy Ham"? I knew Daddy shopped at the organic food mart, but Tiny Pants hadn't even licked my ham for a taste test. He just saw the pieces I had lovingly cut up and dismissed them outright, and with prejudice. When Daddy called the boys that night, I asked him what was so special about his ham.

"It's turkey. He hates turkey, so I tell him it's ham and he eats it," he said.

"But it's not ham, it's turkey."

"But he likes ham."

"No, he doesn't like ham. He likes turkey that you call ham and refuses to eat ham because it is the wrong color. You have to tell him you feed him turkey so I can figure out what he is actually asking me to feed him."

Laughter.

"Daddy's house, Daddy's rules. Good luck with that."

Click.

So from then on we referred to it as "white ham" and "pink ham" and when they finally agreed to try pink ham, they preferred it over white ham, like all good people. However, they complained that some bites were cold and others were warm. I told them that was the way ham was supposed to be, because part of the fun of eating it was the temperature-variable surprise.

ONLY MAMA

HOME | POSTS | ABOUT THIS BLOG | ABOUT ME

My Christmas Peppermint Tray

I don't do Pinterest, for the very simple reason that I know it will eat every spare moment showing me fabulous things that will just make me feel inadequate. I can feel perfectly inadequate on my own, thank you very much.

However, I accidentally got sucked into a Pinterest-type thing this week. I was reading a blog and somehow or another wound up on a page promising that could make my very own peppermint tray. I left the window open for an entire week. I tried to close it, but I couldn't. I was captivated. I needed my own "perfect presentation for Santa's cookies." What kind of mother would I be otherwise?

I could not unsee it. I now knew deep, deep in my bones that my holiday would not be complete unless I made a peppermint tray. Heck, my entire life would not be complete without a peppermint tray. It was my Christmas Destiny.

The directions were pretty simple. Lest you think I am ripping off some poor unsuspecting person's recipe, there are multiple postings of this same or similar recipe all over the internet, so I don't think it's unique to one creator.

Directions
1. Unwrap a lot of candies.
2. Place in a round baking pan lined with tinfoil.
3. Bake for 8 minutes at 350. "Do not walk away . . . make sure the candies do not overmelt."

I unwrapped the candy.

I placed in lined pan.

I put in oven, and checked every 8 seconds for the first minute, then completely forgot about them until the timer went off. Thank God for timers. Now I see why other people are so nuts about them.

I took my creation out of the oven, and it was like a light from Heaven shined down on me. I Made a Freaking Peppermint Tray!

I photographed it, I held it up to the light, I stared at it in wonder. I must repeat: I Made a Freaking Peppermint Tray!

For the rest of the week, I will only answer to Our Lady, Queen of Christmas. So what if I got crappy presents for people? So what if I haven't gotten around to vacuuming yet and the house guests will be here any minute? I made a freaking peppermint tray. My work here is done.

. . . .

Posted by Lara L Monday, December 23, 2013 at 7:28 PM
Labels: Not Necessarily Single, Parenting, Times I Got It Right or Just Got Lucky

Consignment Store Christmas

The same consignment shop that sold me the Halloween costumes saved my ass again at Christmas. I had budgeted one hundred dollars, which sounded like a lot until I went shopping for new toys. Tiny Pants didn't even know it was Christmas, but Big Pants sure as shit did, and that hundred dollars wasn't going to go far at a new toy store.

"Do you have any Thomas trains?" I asked the nice lady behind the counter at the consignment shop. Thomas the Tank Engine was like crack for the preschool set, and Big Pants slept every night with Thomas clutched in one hand and Diesel, Thomas's archnemesis, in the other. I knew that Thomas merchandise got snatched up faster than cookies at a toddler playdate, so I knew my question was likely futile.

"We just got this in—I haven't even put it out yet," the store owner said, hefting a large plastic bin onto the counter. Inside was the complete Thomas Take Along set: twenty-five trains, plenty of snap-together track, Cranky the Crane with working winch, and the smelting yard. "If you take it all, I'll only charge you seventy-five dollars, and I'll throw in the box for free," she said. That left me twenty-five for Tiny Pants, who mainly just wanted to crawl into empty boxes and chew on the dog's tail.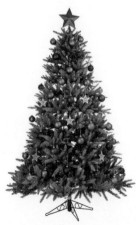

There were so many trains that I had to wrap them in sets of threes and fives. I put some in his stocking and the rest under our little three-foot-tall Christmas tree—Daddy had kept the full-size artificial tree in the divorce, and I couldn't afford a new one. Big Pants got tired of opening presents before he ran out of trains to open, and I had set an impossibly high precedent for Christmases to come.

The next year, I was at the traffic light in front of the same shop and managed to spy Butterscotch the Sit-On Pony in their front window. I had been admiring Butterscotch's twin at Target. It neighed, turned its head, and made loud chewing noises if you stuffed a plastic carrot in its mouth. If Butterscotch the Sit-On Pony had existed when I was a child, it would have been at the top of my Christmas list. I hung a U-ey and went back. That pony must be mine.

When I got home, however, I now had a four-foot-tall horse to hide for the next few weeks and inadequate locations for storage. The Pants brothers' bedroom was in the finished attic. We had converted the basement into a playroom that summer, as it was the coolest place in the house and safest place to do Play-Doh or finger paint. With a lot of effort, I managed to stuff that pony sideways into my closet and tuck it behind my clothes. Unfortunately, I often forgot the pony was in there until I went to get dressed in the morning and opened the door, startling myself in a frightful *Godfather*-type way, only with a stuffed horse head instead of a real one.

ONLY MAMA

HOME | POSTS | ABOUT THIS BLOG | ABOUT ME

Tag-Team Christmas

The best kept secret of single parenting is tag-team Christmas.

My ex and I have an agreement where we both see the kids on Christmas Day, alternating which house they wake up at every other year, and switching at noon. The first year after we separated I prepared myself for the worst Christmas of my life, and my parents agreed to come to support me in what we all thought would be a horrendous outpouring of grief interrupted by a few hours of holiday cheer. We all assumed the crash position and waited for impending negative emotions . . . but they never came.

Here's why:

If you ask my kids, double Christmas is the best part of having two houses. It is the one time of the year when other kids are jealous of them. They get two trees, two stockings, two stops from Santa's sleigh. The kids strike the mother lode twice in the same day, year after year. They are in all their glory, so you get a day off from parental guilt.

But the kids aren't the only ones who benefit. Here's the truth about kids on Christmas—they stay up too late fighting sleep, making it impossible for Santa to come until midnight, and if Santa didn't finish wrapping, Santa might be up until two in the morning. Then the little angels wake up at the crack of dawn, decimate the toy pile in under an hour, and spend the rest of the day whining and being over-sugared and under-slept.

Enter tag-team Christmas. Children wake up at Parent A's house, descend on presents like a pack of hungry hyenas, play with toys for an hour, and just when they start to get to that whiny stage around noon, they get dropped off at Parent B's house. Parent B got to sleep in and finish Santa duty in the morning instead of the middle of the night, so Parent B is not overtired and cranky. Parent A gets to go home and take a nap, and Parent B gets to do Christmas after coffee and breakfast, like a civilized adult.

It is truly a win-win for the parents, and the kids are wallowing around knee-deep in presents, so they're happy, too. Of course, the day-after-Christmas letdown is still unavoidable (heck, I still get it at age forty), but Christmas Day itself is far better when you have someone to tag in with.

· ·

Posted by Lara L Wednesday, December 25, 2013 at 8:27 AM
Labels: Single Parenting, Times I Got It Right or Just Got Lucky

Standing in the Return Line

The fun part of being single is dating. New love is one of the best feelings there is. I haven't ever smoked crack, but people who write psychology articles like to say that new love affects the body much like a drug, though I don't think they actually have firsthand knowledge of what smoking crack feels like, either. In my very limited experience, people who write scholarly articles don't often use illicit street drugs. I tend to think that if they did any drugs, they would be more of the designer preppy drug variety than crack. To be honest, I'm not sure if anyone actually smokes crack anymore. I think it has gone out of fashion, which makes it even less likely that scholarly-article-writing-people smoke crack, at least not habitually. But I digress. The upside of dating is that occasionally you get that falling-in-love happiness where sleep is no longer necessary, and you don't need food to survive—you can live on only one whole wheat cracker and lingering gazes.

The downside of dating is that 90 percent of the time you are not in that mutually falling-in-love state. Sometimes you are falling in love with them, and they are just waiting for someone more preferable to come along. Other times they have fallen in love with you, and you are only keeping them around as a backup plan in case you can't find anyone better. It's not pretty no matter which side of the equation you're on.

I'd like to say that my dating life was a series of dating smart, interesting guys and discovering that we just didn't have that magic spark, so we amicably went our separate ways. That did happen twice, but most of the time dating still had the drama of high school, but with the side benefit of having two tiny children who expected me to pull my shit together, make them breakfast, and not sob uncontrollably on the couch all day.

I felt it was important for my kids not to ever worry about my emotional state, but living in a small house with children who couldn't be trusted out of my sight when there were markers lying about—and there were always markers lying about—made it impossible to go hide in my room. I guess some people—we'll call them aliens—have the type of children who play quietly by themselves without any need for adult interaction, but I didn't have those type of children. If I went into my bedroom, they would stick their little fingers under the door.

"Mama? Mama? What are you doing? Mama? Open the door. Mama? Mama? Mama?" *Suck it up Mama, I need a cookie!* Actually, that's an exaggeration. My kids did love cookies, but not as much as they loved Mama. All they ever wanted was "Mama, Mama, Only Mama!" They wanted to be not just in the same room, but in my lap, or riding on my back around the room like I was their personal pony.

I wanted to be that person, so if my kids caught me crying, I told them I had allergies. If the day was too much to deal with—hours and hours piling up on top of each other, and I needed to text my BFF Asterisk or I was going to suffocate—I took them to the park, or the museum, or anywhere where I could sit on a bench and text while they got to run around and play. If I needed to have a long emotional phone call with my mom, I'd let the boys play in the minivan in the driveway, while I leaned against the side of the vehicle and talked—we could see each other, but they couldn't hear me.

During this time period there were a lot of memes showing up in my Facebook feed about how sad it was that parents were glued to their phones while their precious darlings swung alone on the swing set, and how we only got these moments once in life, and all the selfish moms (like me) who were on our cell phones were going to live a life of regret for not cherishing these moments. Toddler years are best enjoyed in retrospect. When you stay home with little people, day after day, week after week, it's hard to find every moment precious and poignant. I had a personal rule: don't kill the children. Taking care of your emotional needs is necessary to not kill the children. Enjoying the moment is sometimes too much to ask for.

That's not to say that I didn't feel horribly guilty about this—of course I did. At night, when they were asleep, looking all soft and vulnerable and quiet, I hated myself for breaking up their family and then not finding happiness right away. The divorce was supposed to make *someone* happy, so when I wasn't, it all felt very useless. I looked at their sleeping heads, arms, and legs splayed out in uncomfortable-looking positions and wished I had been able to summon more enthusiasm when they were awake. I always resolved to be more present, which meant sometimes I sat on the floor assembling an incredibly long Thomas the Tank Engine track while wearing a Batman costume and telling myself, "Don't cry in front of the children. Don't cry in front of the children."

After the boys were asleep, I sat on my front porch and felt unseen threads connecting me to all the other sleepless single parents out there. I knew there was a whole hidden population just trying to keep themselves together for their children—people who might otherwise give in to depression, anger, or fear, but instead were staring at the same sky I was, just trying to make it one more day, in hopes that somehow, life would get just a little tiny bit easier, and if we could only string together a few slightly easier days, a few more hours of sleep at night, a little less heartbreak, we all might come out okay.

How to Make Fried Dough

One of the major themes of this book is being low-energy, sleep deprived, and overwhelmed most of the time, with a smattering of situational depression thrown in just for fun. The downside of single parenting is that you have no one else to pawn the children off on when you are crabby and the kids are crabby and you really need to get something productive done and they really need you to play Thomas trains. When I got overwhelmed, my first instinct is never to make a color-coded to-do list and tackle my chores one by one until I am filled with a feeling of satisfaction and the kids have clean noses and customized learning-through-play educational plans for the day. Some days, it was hard to summon the wherewithal to leave the house. A lot of times there were things I wanted to do but just couldn't overcome the hypnotically sweet embrace of the sofa.

Like carnivals. Daddy Pants was convinced that carnival rides were completely and totally unsafe and our children should never, ever go on them. Now, I knew that carnival rides were completely and totally fun, but they required abandoning my beloved couch in order to pay way too much money for ride coupons and stand around in the hot sun all day watching my boys go around and around on small boats, cars, or tiny helicopters. However, carnivals have fried dough, and I happen to like fried dough quite a lot. So the decision between standing around in the hot sun versus staying home in my pajamas was much more easily resolved when I learned to make my own fried dough, or at least, a fried-dough-like substance. This isn't the funnel cake variety, but more like what they called "elephant ears" where I came from. I apologize in advance for making you actually use the stove and not the microwave for this one. Sadly, fried dough requires hot oil, and I have yet to figure out how to do this in a microwave. I'll keep trying, though.

Cautionary note: If you are like me and have placed a large wooden cutting board over the top of your stove in order to increase counter space, you must completely remove it for this recipe. I tried to just push the cutting board to one side of the stove, revealing one front and one rear burner, but it turns out that does not provide enough distance between the burner and the cutting board, even though it looks like it will all work out just fine. Also, wooden cutting boards are flammable, or at least scorch-able. Even if you agree with me that a slightly scorched cutting board has more character than a plain board with no interesting backstory, you will be forced to repeatedly answer embarrassing questions from people (usually men) who don't understand how easy it is to set a cutting board on fire.

Ingredients
Vegetable oil, canola oil, whatever "regular" unfancy oil
    you generally use
1 tube/can of biscuits
powdered sugar

Procedure
1. Heat oil in frying pan. How much? Like half an inch deep. Heat until it is hot, but not smoking.
2. Take biscuits out of can/tube and stretch them out until they are double their original size.
3. Place pulled biscuit dough carefully into hot oil, trying not to splatter your arms, because that shit hurts. The rule about never frying bacon naked is applicable here as well.

4. The first one will give you a good idea of how long to wait before you flip them. You don't really want them brown, more like dark blond. And you only want to flip them once, because the more you flip them, the oiler they get. So sort of lift one up with a spatula and peek underneath. When it gets to that dark blond color, flip carefully.

5. Place on paper-towel-lined plate to soak up the oil, you know, like you do with bacon.

6. Sprinkle liberally with powdered sugar, flip over, and sprinkle other side with powdered sugar.

7. Don't forget to turn off the stove, because yikes—that could go poorly.

8. Alternatively, you can skip the powdered sugar and spread with butter and jelly. Try it once, as an experiment. Even though powdered sugar seems to be the only appropriate way to go, butter and jelly is a very fine way to eat fried dough as well, and who always has powdered sugar in their cabinet? Aliens, that's who.

Male Friends, With and Without Benefits

When Tiny Pants turned two, I was having one of those endlessly long days of just trying not to cry in front of the children. I had broken up with my boyfriend, or was still in the negotiation process of breaking up with my boyfriend, I can't exactly remember which now. Daddy Pants was taking the Pants brothers to Chicago the next day—I was not going to see my precious little Tiny Pants on his actual birthday. Luckily, he couldn't read a calendar yet, so he didn't actually know what day his birthday really was, though I sure as shit did. I decorated the dining room with balloons and streamers, wrapped presents, and baked a cake. I tried not to think about my babies going out of town for a week without me. I tried not to think about the boyfriend drama. I had to save the party, so I invited over my friend Herman.

I met Herman through Asterisk. He lived a mile and a half away, and though he was single, he was not a love match. Herman was the one guy I knew who actually meant it when he said he wanted to be friends. We hung out often both when I had the kids and when they were at Daddy Pants's house.

The kids loved Herman, and since Herman had no kids of his own, he was always willing to let them jump on his head. He had a fake leg, and he'd turn it a full 360 degrees to entertain them. He was generally laughing and he had the kids convinced that he was really a pirate. On Tiny Pants's second birthday, when I couldn't smile and felt like a hollowed-out husk of sadness, Herman came over with a three-foot-tall pink stuffed bunny (because he liked to find the most obnoxious/irritating gift he could find) and ate cake with us. He took the pressure off, as the kids were so excited to see him, they no longer noticed if I was smiling or not.

• • •

About a year after becoming single, I got into an exciting relationship with a man, and at his urging, we exchanged house keys after about six weeks. I had stayed in touch with the very first person to take me out, back the very first week I was single. He was an amazing person and also lived several states away, and I have never seen him again in real life. This was actually pretty cool, because that first week I needed a date to prove that it was possible to find someone smart and interesting and also single, but I didn't need an actual boyfriend in town distracting me from settling into my new life. We used to talk on the phone every few days, which drifted to every week, then to once a month as our conversations naturally progressed from talking about trying to meet up again to trading anecdotes about people we were dating in the real world.

I told First Date Friend about this new guy I had been seeing lately. He was very nice and also had a kid who was just a couple of years older than Big Pants. His daughter made him sandwiches for lunch when she was at his house, and wrote his name on his lunch bag in marker. First Date Friend interrupted what I can now see was a very dull story and asked, "Is he endlessly fascinating? Are you just dying to hear what will come out of his mouth next?"

"Well, no," I had to admit.

"Yeah, who needs that?" First Date Friend replied. Suddenly I looked at my new boyfriend and realized that I was settling. Within a week, we had broken up and I needed my key back.

Getting a key back isn't that big of a deal if you don't have kids, but for me, the potential consequences of giving the wrong person a key to my house were terrifying. I got my key back, but called Herman, who came over the next day—luckily it was his day off—and changed my locks for me, just in case the boyfriend had kept a copy. I learned to keep my keys to myself after that. All I could think about were my two sweet boys, who weren't even tall enough to turn the dead bolt or dial 911. What would happen to them if someone broke in? I didn't want to turn into a Lifetime TV movie. Nothing happened, but I was aware that I was one bad decision away from a colossal mistake. I realized I wasn't ready for a relationship. As much as I wanted to run from my loneliness, I had an obligation to stand still for a little while and wait for my inner storm to subside.

That sounds so good and grown-up, doesn't it? But my decision not to become involved didn't mean that I wanted to stop having sex. I had spent a grand total of fifteen years in consecutive monogamous relationships with men who didn't particularly want to have sex with me. My skin was starved for touch, so although I stopped looking for a relationship, I ventured into the world of friends with benefits. Unfortunately, I was incapable of separating the physical from the emotional. I was a girl who always became attached, even when I didn't want to.

UnobtainiMan

I found the television remote and turned off the overhead light. The TV's glow turned my small burnt-orange bedroom cave-like. Just beyond my double bed the shadows obscured the books, papers, and who knew what-all that was piled on my desk, as well as the scattered clothing on the floor, making the room seem neater. I made a nest of my throw pillows, pulled my mushy-soft blue blanket over my shoulder, and folded my lover's old T-shirt in my hands, tucking it next to my face. On my nightstand was the lava lamp, red oil and glitter swirling and dancing above the bulb at the base. I left it on all night long.

I had not loved a bedroom so much since I was a child. When I moved in, the bottom half of the walls had been a gray sand texture and the top an icy pink. A year later, Asterisk and I glazed my bedroom walls by hand— she used red and I used yellow, backtracking and overlaying the two colors until we had many brushy orange tones. Our decision not to prep ahead of time left a sloppy, unfinished line halfway up the walls where the sand texture below met the smooth walls above. To cover up our shoddy job, I created a border of photographs, old ticket stubs, postcards, mementos, and all the odds and ends I had been carrying around in a shoebox for a decade.

It was here that UnobtainiMan and I learned the language of each other's skin, emboldened by whiskey and desire postponed too long. We stretched our stolen interludes as long as we could—an hour turning to two and then three.

But of course it wasn't that simple. Although he had no children, he was still legally married.

My last relationship had ended with my boyfriend saying, "You were an empty whore when I met you, now you're just a lying whore." Until I could work out why my relationships so often turned septic, I didn't need another boyfriend. Yet I did not want to be abstinent. All of my ex-husband's recriminations of *no, not now, don't start that* had left me feeling undesired, unfulfilled, and indecent in my wanting. I craved caresses and being drunk on the scent of another person's skin. I wanted to never again be told that I was too much—too needy, too sexual, too *me*. Dating someone who was still entangled and therefore not capable of moving in or spending the night seemed like a reasonable compromise.

We had met online, but after a year of people shopping, I was worn out with it. Instead of sending some sort of self-promotional-yet-flirty message, I sent him an essay. He read it and saw who I was inside the words, without a shell of social nicety. My intention of remaining friends with benefits was quickly a lot more complicated than I thought it would be. Casual intimacy turned out to be something neither of us was capable of. Within a few weeks, it was too late to pretend we were not in love in spite of his messy and unresolved marital situation. Love as in *torment*. Love as in *wretched yearning*. Of course, I should have known it was a bad idea. I had never been able to love half-heartedly.

Yet I needed him to go. I did not want this liaison to swallow me. I needed to tend to the boys first. I needed to finish my schoolwork and find time to write the stories rattling around my head. I had a long history of allowing relationships to turn me into someone with neither opinions nor passion of my own. I needed him to leave so that I could keep track of who I wanted to become. I didn't introduce him to my friends, didn't invite him over when my parents were in town. Some weeks felt perfectly balanced, others not so much. People thought I was strong and independent—I knew how often I was neither. Still, I didn't need to create a new family for the Pants brothers. I needed to learn that just the three of us were enough.

• • •

We did one thing right. We started our affair with our skin removed. "What are you most ashamed of?" he asked me that first day on the porch, and I decided to tell him. He didn't laugh or flinch so I said more, and he matched my stories with his own humiliations and regrets. "Tell me something true," I implored one night, two weeks after we met. He told me the story of his biggest childhood shame. We both carried gnarled scars from marriages to people we loved but who seemed repulsed by physical intimacy with us. We discussed our childhoods, and the big and small ways we were failed by our parents. We discussed past lovers and past sexual escapades, and I did not feel like a whore. We all have that one fantasy, the one that we can't speak of to anyone, because it seems too weird or reveals too much of our shadow selves. When I mustered the nerve to say mine aloud, he did not spit on the ground like Daddy Pants had. Instead, my lover said, "We can try that."

Our conversations weren't only confessional. We talked about dreams, childhood pets, and the things we were most proud of. He explained how ants communicated, how sine waves worked, and he read every essay and story I wrote. I could tell when they were good, because then he'd get lost in the sentences and stop correcting my verb tenses. If they hadn't gelled yet, we talked about what stopped the reader short, what made sense only in my brain. He sent me music: lyrics he was writing, versions of instrumental tracks that expressed his feelings without words. We saw each other's scars, stretch marks, and insecurities, and we did not look away in disgust. For the first time, I looked in the mirror and cherished everything that made me different. It was because of, not in spite of, my flaws that I was beautiful, worthwhile.

• • •

My love life was thorny and existed only in shadows, but it made me live as a single woman, solving my problems myself, learning to do things on my own. Because I was in love with this unobtainable person, I wasn't spending energy on a finding a boyfriend, and I could focus on my children and my own dreams.

School

When I left Daddy Pants, I had an associate's degree in liberal arts and a fine collection of student loans I accumulated by starting and dropping out of many institutions of higher learning. After the kids were born, I broached the subject with Daddy Pants of going back to school yet again, only this time to major in creative writing. He was decidedly not enthusiastic. It wasn't going to happen without a major tussle, and I didn't know how to form words with my mouth that said, "This is important to me." Instead I said, "Okay, I don't need to go." Instead of giving up on school, I gave up on the relationship.

• • •

After a year of being on my own I wanted to go back to school and finish that degree. I had always wanted to be a writer—all the way back to high school when I wrote exceedingly bad rhyming poetry—but I didn't think I had a story to tell. When I was pregnant with Tiny Pants, I was suddenly flooded with stories—I wrote more than four hundred pages in my last trimester. This was what I wanted to do with my life, even if it wasn't practical and even if there was no money in it. I had already prioritized passion over practicality when I left Daddy Pants.

• • •

I started applying to schools based solely on their name and reputation, eventually choosing one because a guy I once dated liked it. I sent back my acceptance and deposit without actually perusing the course catalog or knowing how much financial aid I qualified for. It turned out not to be the best way to choose a school, and I stopped dating that guy before fall semester started, so I couldn't even impress him with my scholastic achievement. I discovered that the school wasn't conveniently located, nor was it designed for adult learners with jobs, and that financial aid wasn't going to be as much as I had hoped, but I didn't learn any of these things until after I was already enrolled. My boss allowed me to manipulate my schedule around classes, but since our office was only open 9–5, it involved a lot of scurrying between school and work during the day. As soon as I got involved in a project at work, it was time to drop it and drive to class. When I came back, I needed forty-five minutes to find my place again. Eventually I found myself sobbing in my minivan in the school parking lot, unable to go to class because I felt my paper wasn't good enough to turn in. That was the end of that, except, of course, for the $9,000 in additional student loans.

The next time I went back to school—two years later—I did a lot of research first. I knew exactly how much time and money it was going to cost, and I took all online classes. I carried my books or e-reader to the playground, or upstairs to the kids' bedroom. I learned that I couldn't write much of anything when they were awake, but I could deflect errant stuffed animals whizzing by my head while reading. After they were asleep, I dragged my laptop to the front porch to do my writing, where the cold kept me awake long enough to finish my assignments. This time, I didn't drop out.

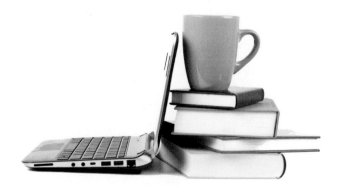

HOME | POSTS | ABOUT THIS BLOG | ABOUT ME

In Which I Am Forced to Commune with Nature in a Foot of Snow and Write a Bad Poem About It

I am taking creative writing, which is great. I have been dying to take creative writing since I returned to college. However, I became less excited about it when I was told that I had to go out into the woods and be still with nature and write a poem about it.

I like to think my teacher did not anticipate the discomfort of sitting in snow in the winter when she crafted this assignment; I assume it was a more temperate day or she lives in Florida, or something rational. Or perhaps she has a malevolent streak—I'm not sure yet, it is only the second day of class.

However, I am committed to my writing so I took a plastic Walmart folding chair into the snow and sat on it. My bum was a mere inch above the snow, but luckily, it wasn't an aggressive-chair-climbing-bum-attacking kind of snow. The snow stayed right where it was, one inch below my posterior. I looked at snow and thought poetic thoughts. I looked very closely at the snow. I noted how the sparkle was burning my retinas. I wrote poetic thoughts:

> I brought to the woods, a folding chair
> because the snow was deep.

I looked up, and what was looking right back at me? A deer? No. A rabbit, skunk, squirrel, chipmunk, or bear? None of those, either. It was a trail cam. You know, one of those things hunters and nature enthusiasts put in the woods to take pictures of wildlife. Great, I went to the woods to be alone, and now I can't even wipe my nose on my sleeve without someone watching. Not that I would ever do that, obviously.

I looked down. Inside my footprints were lots of specks. I would venture a disproportionate number of brown specks in white footprints in the middle of nowhere. I looked at my boots. They did not appear muddy. I suddenly remembered someone once said something about snow fleas, or was it snow lice? I put my head down to investigate, but seeing as I didn't know if they were actual bugs or not, I didn't know if they jumped. I decided not to look to closely. I tried again to think poetically.

> I brought to the woods a folding chair
> because the snow was deep
> the animals were hibernating
> the bears were all asleep
> from a branch the snow did fall
> my poem sucks big donkey balls.

I gave up and spent the rest of the day at an outdoor bonfire drinking adult beverages and making tiny snowmen because I was feeling creative but too lazy to get up and make a full-sized snowperson.

I actually spent several days working on my bad snow poem trying to improve it, and I think I finally did. It is probably the longest I ever worked on a poem, especially one I did not care anything about.

No, you voyeurs, I'm not printing my finished poem here, unless you comment a lot and request me to, because then you could secretly ridicule my poem in your heads but I would get page views out of it, and page views stroke my ego and make me feel warm and fuzzy, so it would balance out.

(continued)

Postscript

I am including the final poem I turned in, because it seems unkind to be so withholding. It's not a great poem, and I promise not to subject you to more lame poetry, but since the art of memoir is about honesty and not trying to look smarter, hipper, or artier on the page than in real life, I am giving you my wishy-washy poem, lest you harbor any hopes that I am secretly a great poet. I'm not.

Final Poem

Skeletal stillness of bare branches
against white on darker white of snow
Hard angled ice chips dance in sunlight
Childhood sidewalks
Of soft sparkling quartz

snow falls from a branch
no wind to provoke it
or animal chatter to explain
it falls because it must;
it is destined to fall from the moment
it chose to rest on this branch
villainous sun disturbing its rest, warming it, enticing it

Slide, it says,
Give up your intolerable peace
join your companion snow below
remain in the gray shadows
without a hint of brown, or glacial cerulean
the sun cannot reach you here
to disturb your peace or make you sparkle

. . . .

Posted by Lara L Friday, January 11, 2013 at 9:44 AM
Labels: Grown Up Time

In Which I Go Out to Eat Alone and Live to Tell About it

I'm very good at doing big things, like leaving husbands, finding jobs, or flying across the country on my own. What I couldn't do was go to a restaurant by myself. It was the little things about going somewhere new that bogged me down—where to park, what to wear, what door to go in, and whether to choose a booth or table. If I thought about the little things too much, I couldn't leave the house at all. I had several girlfriends talk me through scary things, like finding the right door to go into for a ballet class at the high school, or where to park to go to the Science Center for the first time. In front of the children I was mostly able to force myself to be brave and venture forth. Anxiety can be contagious, and I didn't want the Pants brothers to catch it. As it was, they were afraid of bees and going on playdates without me. If they knew that going new places terrified me, they'd never make it through kindergarten, and I desperately needed them to go to kindergarten someday. Although I was brave in front of the children, when I was on my own, fear paralyzed me. I had to stop dragging my married girlfriends along every time I wanted to go out.

UnobtainiMan told me to take myself out to dinner on one especially low night. I was absolutely terrified by the idea. He suggested Don's Lighthouse—a white-linen restaurant that was out of my price range, but he promised he'd pay if I could successfully eat there.

"What do I wear?" I asked him.

"Like what someone would wear to work," he replied, which didn't really help, because I wore jeans and T-shirts to my job, and I knew that wasn't what he meant. Plus, it was cold out, and I didn't want to freeze. I wasn't above freezing to look cute, mind you, but I was going somewhere alone with no one to appreciate my cuteness. It was a waste of goose bumps. I settled on slacks and a white sweater. I didn't feel especially adorable, but I looked tall and lanky, and lanky felt like an accomplishment. I couldn't manage sexy, but I could do tall reasonably well.

"Just go and sit at the bar and order a spring salad with a steak on top," he advised.

I drove to the restaurant. I asked to be seated at the bar. I looked at the menu. There was only a winter salad and it did not come with steak. This might not seem like that big of a deal to anyone else. In fact, it doesn't seem like that big of a deal to me in retrospect, but at the time, my eyes prickled with tears and if I hadn't already ordered (but not yet paid for) a glass of wine I would have left. I couldn't do this.

"My friend said the spring salad is really good here," I said to the bartender, who had so far been ignoring me as much as humanly possible—she obviously could sense my desperation for human contact.

"It's winter. We have winter salad because it is winter," she explained like I was a toddler. Admittedly, I knew that this was a stupid thing to get hung up on. I wanted to tell her that although it was freezing out it was actually March and therefore spring salad was seasonally appropriate, because I had an urgent need to correct the injustice of it, but instead I meekly ordered the winter salad and asked if I could have a steak cut up on top. This was also a problem for the bartender. She insisted the steak had to come on a separate plate and I would have to do any required cutting on my own. Seeing as how I cut up meat for myself and children every freaking day, I knew I had the skills required for the job, but I was getting pissed at UnobtainiMan for suggesting that I order something that did not exist. I realize that I could have just looked at the menu and ordered something else and avoided all this hassle, but:

1. I didn't expect it to be such a big deal,
2. UnobtainiMan had promised to reimburse me if I successfully went out to eat alone, and I didn't want to run up too big of a tab, and
3. Anxiety isn't rational in any way, shape, or form.

I ordered the winter salad with a side of un-cut-up steak. Of course, the inevitable happened—the food came, and I cut the steak all by myself and ate it. It wasn't a big deal at all. An older man sat down at the bar next to me, and we wound up talking about insurance—he was an agent, I used to be in the business before I had children. We had more wine and discussed both of our divorces. At the end of the night he offered me a job, which I didn't take, but appreciated the offer. I tipped the bartender 40 percent to prove to her that I belonged in fancy restaurants. I think in retrospect that such a large tip kind of proved that I wasn't comfortable in fancy restaurants, but I wanted her to feel guilty for being so difficult. Unfortunately, she never reported back if this triggered her guilt or not.

• • •

After that first night, I often stopped at my favorite restaurant on the way home from work—not Don's Lighthouse, but The Melt, a funky place with a lot of light-up plastic yard ornaments and cheese sandwiches the size of my head. I sat at the bar and talked to whomever else was eating alone—there were always plenty of single diners. It no longer seemed so intimidating. After a few months, I couldn't believe I had ever thought going to eat by myself was too scary or lonely to contemplate.

• • •

The Melt is known for their cheesy sandwiches on homemade bread. I can't possibly replicate the divine greasy goodness that is a Melt sandwich, but I can make the world's easiest beer bread, and you can melt cheese on it (because why not?) and that is pretty divine and in keeping with the spirit of The Melt. It is so easy that children can make it, except that you probably shouldn't encourage children to open beer bottles unsupervised.

The World's Simplest Beer Bread

Ingredients

1 bottle or can of beer, any variety or age. I generally
   have a bottle or two of beer in my fridge that someone
   left behind, and since I don't drink beer the lone bottle
   rattles around my fridge for many months or even years.
   This doesn't matter. Beer drinkers may have rules about
   warm beer or old beer, but for these purposes, as long
   as it still makes that *fzzzz* noise when you open it, it's
   fine. My personal favorite for beer bread is hard cider,
   because I bought a six-pack two years ago and no one
   has any interest in drinking it. It adds sweetness. Summer
   Shandy adds lemoniness. Regular beer is perfectly
   adequate at making the magic happen. Some people
   say that beer bread can be made with any nonalcoholic
   carbonated beverage, but I haven't tried it because if I
   have a Sprite or ginger ale I'm drinking it. I have no other
   good use for beer.

3 cups of instant pancake mix (the just-add-water kind).
   Pay attention: this part is important. You are supposed
   to sift the pancake mix to avoid creating a bread-shaped
   brick, but I am not the type of person who owns a sifter.
   However, if you pour the measured mix slowly into the
   bowl and fluff it up with a whisk as you pour it, it works
   out just fine. If you don't have a whisk—or don't have
   a clean whisk—a fork will work as well. If you child is
   assisting you in this endeavor keep an eye on them
   because pancakes mix flies in a way many small children
   find satisfying.

1 serving of ⅓ cup of butter and 1 serving of ¼ cup butter.
   I mean two individual servings of butter, melted in the

microwave. You can use one measuring cup and refill it. It may seem excessive, but have you ever said *this has too much butter*? No, you have not.

Procedure
1. Add beer to the fluffed-up pancake mix.
2. Add ⅓ cup melted butter. Stir. Pour into greased bread pan. If you don't have a bread pan, you can pour it into a round cake pan/pie pan. (Actually, I always make it in a round cake pan. While I assume it will work in a bread pan I haven't actually tried it since I don't own one.) Pour ¼ cup of butter over the dough.
3. I advise placing a piece of tinfoil at the bottom of the oven to catch any drips, because when the bread rises sometimes the butter overflows. I think most people besides me already knew to do this.
4. Bake at 375 for 50 minutes to 1 hour. (When the edge pulls away from the side and gets brown it is done.)

BUT WAIT. What if you've happened to find the man of your dreams and by chance they are upstairs in your bedroom right now and you have nothing in your kitchen to feed them, and like my stepmother, cooking is part of your man-trapping strategy (see "Swedish Meatballs") and you have (bizarrely) turned to me to help solve your problems? Or, what if it is morning and there is no man in the house but you are hungry and in great need of a breakfast treat and just happened to read this far and all the talk of beer bread is making you want carbs but not just bread carbs but something more fun? No worries, I got you.

Beer Bread Breakfast Muffins

(The word "muffin" is a little misleading. They're more like small portable breakfast breads. Muffin implies a sweetness that requires adding at least ½ cup of sugar.)

Procedure

1. Crank up that oven to 400 because it's probably a weekday and you have to get to work.
2. Make batter as above.
3. Take a big overflowing handful of mixed nuts from the can and seal the nuts in a ziplock bag. Bash them to smithereens with a saucepan or other heavy item. (I do this on the floor.) Note: if there really is a new man waiting upstairs, you might want to check for nut allergies before proceeding so you don't kill him accidentally. If your hands are as gargantuan as mine, this results in around ½ cup of smashed nuts.
4. Add 2 boxes of raisins. If you choose to buy raisins in the more economical large round container, aim for ½ cup.
5. Add 1 tablespoon of cinnamon and ½ teaspoon vanilla.
6. If you didn't have hard cider and used regular beer, I'd add a small handful of brown sugar to the mix, or maybe sprinkle sugar on top.
7. Spray muffin tin with nonstick cooking spray. Scoop batter into the muffin cups. Bake for 20 minutes. Serve warm and with butter.

Remember, *and this is important:* if he really is the love of your life and if the muffins are a complete fail, it won't matter. One True Loves will find morning-after muffin fails endearing.

First Day of School

Big Pants started kindergarten. The very first day, I dressed him in a white polo and uniform navy blue shorts. Daddy Pants came over to take photos before school. I couldn't believe I was trusting some unknown teacher to take care of my little boy for seven hours. What if he needed a snack? Was he allowed a snack? Should I pack a snack? Seeing as there was no snack guidance, I packed one anyway, completely unsure that he would even remember its location in his backpack—he wouldn't turn five years old until a month after school started. He looked so small walking into the brick building with his socks pulled up to his knees.

I did what any good and reasonable mother would do. I played with Tiny Pants in the morning, then I took a long and delicious nap when Tiny Pants went to sleep. Kindergarten was a very, very good idea. After school, Big Pants's teacher delivered him to my car personally. She had on lots and lots of glittery green eyeshadow and a really cool and funky necklace. I wanted her to adopt me.

"I'm sorry about his shirt," she said. Big Pants's white shirt was covered in pink smudges. "We had a fruit roll-up incident at lunch."

"I tried to unwrap my fruit roll-up and it got stuck to my shirt," Big Pants explained.

"It took all of lunch to unstick him," she expanded. I thanked her and buckled Big Pants into his booster seat.

"So what else did you eat today?" I asked Big Pants on the way home.

"I told you, a fruit roll-up," he answered. I must have heard wrong—my child ate every fifteen minutes all day long.

"But what else?" I asked.

"Nothing. That was the first thing I tried to eat. Then lunch was over."

I have never felt more of a failure as a mother then that moment—I had betrayed him with my foolish lunch choices. Luckily, he didn't hold it against me, as he was too excited about the kids he sat next to, the games they played, and the books they read. Big Pants was making his way in the world, fruit roll-up mishaps or no.

ONLY MAMA

HOME | POSTS | ABOUT THIS BLOG | ABOUT ME

The Tooth Fairy Fell Asleep

Yesterday Big Pants lost his third tooth. I didn't see it happen (I was in the bathroom) but it involved couch wrestling and a blanket and his brother and then the tooth was out.

The losing of teeth is a big deal in these parts. We have a special box for the tooth with a fairy on it. Big Pants always writes a note to the tooth fairy asking to keep his tooth, an idea stolen from a classmate. Tiny Pants was so jealous that I thought he might take pliers to his own teeth, so the tooth fairy and I had a little discussion, and now he gets a lollipop under his pillow when his brother loses a tooth. You know, to rot his teeth out faster. Except when the tooth fairy goes to sleep and forgets to come.

Two little boys in great distress woke me up to tell me that the tooth fairy had forgotten them, and maybe she didn't really exist.

ARRRRRGGGHHHH! Think, Mama, think!

I knew the tooth fairy was supposed to come. I even made sure to get singles because the tooth fairy cannot ever leave a $20. And then I went to sleep. I was even sober, for those wondering. I was just really tired. I didn't even make it until 10:00 p.m. to see the end of my show.

Those sweet boys looked at me, and all on their own came up with the idea that maybe she left clues for a treasure hunt. I looked at

(continued)

the clock. 6:52 a.m. They are not allowed to wake me before 7:00 a.m, so I sternly sent them back upstairs for eight minutes.

———————————————————

Eight minutes, eight minutes, eight minutes.

I ran downstairs to find my purse . . . which I had left in the car, which was parked outside in a detached garage with a loud door. I was never gonna make that happen secretly in eight minutes. No, six minutes left.

I dug through my change bowl and found eight quarters, which I put in an envelope, on which I wrote, "It was too heavy to carry upstairs." I hid the envelope under the couch pillow. Ran to the kitchen and found a lollipop—not in a good flavor, but still, a lollipop nonetheless. That went under the pillow on the other side of the couch. I ran back upstairs and into my room, just in time.

The boys appeared, telling me of the clues they found in their room. (God only knows what clues, seeing as I hadn't left any.) We decided to start the coffeepot (my idea), then we would all look around downstairs. They found more clues in the living room (a messy house provides many clues through the random distribution of objects, like pennies on the floor and a stray feather and a hat that hadn't been seen in over a year. If you clean your house regularly, you are missing out on this possible lifesaving clue-providing miracle I was afforded this morning).

I yelled at them to fix the pillows on the couch, and get whatever that was under there off the cushions. My house may be chaotic, but I like to have a clean sofa, so this wasn't too weird of a request, I think. Lo and behold, the tooth fairy's surprise was found. Phew!

There was some letdown, because quarters aren't as cool as dollars, and some confusion about what the signs they had discovered meant, and why the tooth fairy didn't have dollar bills. But the tooth fairy came. That's what matters, right?

"At least we have proof that the tooth fairy really exists," I overheard one of the beastie boys say to the other.

(Yet again, I must say phew.)

. . . .

Posted by Lara L Saturday, January 19, 2013 at 7:46 AM
Labels: Not My Finer Moments

The Big Wheel

I have always been a big fan of over-the-top birthdays. Buying toys for your kids is almost like going back in time and buying them for your child-self. Plus, there's always a measure of guilt for the divorce which drives my need to make every damn occasion the best thing that ever happened in their life. But there's also the complication of not having a whole shit-ton of money to accomplish the over-the-topness previously mentioned.

It turned out that a big, red, shiny, new Big Wheel was the lowest price gift with the biggest wow factor I could come up with for Tiny Pants's third birthday. UnobtainiMan—who had no children of his own, I might add—insisted that Tiny Pants would never be able to reach the pedals, but I read the specs and the seat was adjustable. Besides, I had ridden my very own Big Wheel when I was his age. I remembered pulling the brake handle—which only stopped one rear wheel—and sliding triumphantly across the driveway. I remembered trying to pedal in gravel and the front wheel spinning uselessly. I remembered the blue plastic storage compartment behind the seat that was very useful for carrying special things like dried-out frog carcasses. I was not going to be dissuaded.

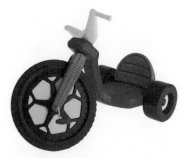

I went to Toys "R" Us and purchased one box of Big Wheel. I couldn't afford the additional assembly fee, but I figured that assembling a Big Wheel wouldn't be that hard. I figured wrong.

I waited for the boys to go to their father's house the week of the birthday before I opened the box. An assembled Big

Wheel seemed like a large item to have to hide, so I needed to wait till the last minute. I dragged the box into the middle of my bedroom floor and opened it. I found the directions. In an attempt to be universally understood, they had no words, only pictures and arrows. Unfortunately, I'm not the kind of girl who is good with pictures and arrows. I am the kind of girl who is good with words and also needs a lot of reassurance and encouragement to assemble anything. Still, I laid out the pieces. I looked at the diagrams. I practiced deep breathing. I put the wheels together and attached the pedals and seat, then discovered that I had an extra part. I don't mean I had an extra part as in a screw or bolt or whatever. I understand that manufacturers occasionally give people a few extras of these items because they assume people like me will drop the baggie on the floor and scatter the hardware all over, and that people like me may also suck at housekeeping and therefore don't have a neat and tidy bedroom to make it possible to find the scattered wing nuts, so they give us a few to spare. I am talking about a large blue plastic part that is very definitely not a spare anything seeing as it was the only large blue plastic part in the box of that approximate shape and size.

UnobtainiMan was out of town, and although he couldn't help me, he got to be on the receiving end of a phone call in which I held him personally responsible for the Big Wheel assembly failure, as he was the closest thing I had to a boyfriend, and Big Wheel assembly seemed like something that fell into boyfriend territory. He kept insisting that I was smart and capable and if I only calmed down I would be able to do it. I found this slightly less than helpful. I didn't want to do it. I wanted to watch him do it.

Since I knew that I was an utter failure at Big Wheel assembly and the birthday was going to happen whether the Big Wheel was assembled or not, and since I also knew that there was no money for a replacement Large and Impressive Present, I threw myself on the mercy of my friend Herman.

Herman was a mechanic and could fix anything. I was sure he would find the Big Wheel easy to assemble. What I didn't anticipate was how hysterical Herman would find my meltdown. He laughed on the phone when I begged him for help. When he saw the pieces all over my bedroom floor, he laughed so hard I could see his back teeth (which were very white). And he laughed when I showed him the despicable diagram.

"It's an extra part," He explained.

"It can't be an extra part," I insisted.

"It's an alternate assembly, if you don't want to install the hand brake."

"But there is extra space on the axle!" I wept.

Herman kept laughing as he tightened down the screws. Miraculously, everything snapped magically into place.

The next day, Tiny Pants was super excited to pull the sheet off of the red and blue Big Wheel. He sat on the seat, and just like UnobtainiMan predicted, his feet didn't reach the pedals. He liked to sit on it while watching TV, though, and eventually he grew into it.

Experimental Mama Cooking: Congealed S'more Stew

I like to do my experimental Mama cooking when there are no witnesses. One day while the kids were at school I was both hungry and wanted an excuse to avoid cleaning the house. I had all the makings for s'mores from a failed cookout and a new dishwasher. It seemed like the perfect way to test the new dishwasher was to make something as sticky as possible.

Ingredients

2 tablespoons of butter, divided

Half a bag of marshmallows that had sort of half-melted several months ago and now were a sticky marshmallow conglomeration

2 Hershey bars

Somewhere around 10 graham crackers

Procedure

1. I first melted 1 tablespoon of butter in a pan over medium heat because it seemed like it might keep things from sticking.
2. Next, I added half a bag of stuck-together marshmallows.

(continued)

3. I broke up two candy bars and threw them in pan while stirring.
4. Then, I crumbled up graham crackers into bite-size pieces and stirred that in as well.
5. It looked sticky, so I added another tablespoon of butter even though I was intending to save the rest of the butter for morning toast so I wouldn't have to go to the store. This appeared to be the right decision. Stirring. Did I mention you should stir this frequently? Stir. Don't leave the room. Don't eat a snack. Stir. When it looks melted, turn off the stove.

It occurred to me that this concoction should be cooled on wax paper, so I went to Tiny Pants's art room as this was the last place I remembered seeing it. No joy. I briefly wondered if I should try using a brown paper bag to cool the goop on, but that seemed imprudent, so instead I sprayed a plate with cooking spray and dumped the melted gooey mass onto it and put it in the fridge to cool. Cooling seemed necessary because at this point my experiment could only be eaten with a spoon and determination. However, a repairman came so I forgot to put on a timer or anything practical like that. I checked it after what felt like twenty minutes because I needed more coffee, and the coffee pot and the refrigerator are in the same room. The chocolate was hardening but there were several globs of marshmallow that didn't get stirred in properly that appeared as if they would never achieve anything approaching a solid state, so I closed the fridge door and waited longer. After the repairman left (maybe an hour later) I checked again and it had coagulated. I cut it up into pieces and ate one. The cooking spray made them a little greasy on the bottom, but also kept them from sticking to the plate. I ate another and then counted how many pieces remained, and since there was now an odd number of treats and I have an even number of children, I ate a third. They are surprisingly light and airy for being an artery death wad of sugary goo.

I filled the pot with dish soap and warm water right before the repairman arrived, and this magically melted off all the sticky residue from the pot, so I didn't get to test my new dishwasher after all.

The Mama Contract

When I got pregnant with Big Pants, I told Daddy Pants that he was going to be responsible for discipline, because our raising two dogs together had already proven that I was incapable of such things. After we divorced, it became readily apparent that I would need to learn some skills, and quickly.

Daddy Pants tried to help by teaching me his patented death look.

"Stare at the kids like you want to rip their heads off. This only works if you actually want to rip their heads off."

I tried his death-stare technique, but I couldn't compete with the Teletubbies/Elmo/dancing puppets that were on the TV 24/7. The kids just looked away and avoided my death stare altogether. Some people might think turning off the TV would have been better parenting, but how else was I ever going to pour a cup of coffee, comb my hair, or change the baby's diaper without Tiny Pants escaping to gleefully run butt-naked throughout the downstairs? The television was my co-parent. Don't worry, we only watched PBS or the DVDs I forgot to return the library because I was too poor for cable.

The programs we watched (seeing as we had no Nickelodeon or Disney Channel) can be summed up into four general categories:

1. Cartoons and other new forms of animation I don't know the word for
2. Gay Men
3. Puppets
4. Gay Men with Puppets

So really, it wasn't nearly as scarring as CNN or something.

Anyway, the death stare didn't work for me, and I just didn't have the stomach for harsh punishments, thanks to Divorce Guilt. Mostly, I survived on threats and bribes, until I discovered the Mama Contract.

I told my children that all mothers were required to sign the Mama Contract before they could take their babies home from the hospital. It clearly spells out all rules Mamas have to follow when raising children, such as:

1. Only one child can cry at a time. Whomever is crying first wins—the second child must wait until the first child is done crying before they can begin. (This actually works!)
2. No Jell-O in the living room.
3. You can't have cake for breakfast.
4. No farting on people's heads. Especially Mama's.

Whenever the kids complained about something completely unreasonable that I asked them to do, such as wearing two matching shoes or not going outside naked, I could tell them, "Don't blame me, it's the Mama Contract. I don't make the rules—I only enforce them." They still believe this is an actual thing, and I'm not telling them otherwise.

ONLY MAMA

HOME | POSTS | ABOUT THIS BLOG | ABOUT ME

Homework Avoidance

There is nothing like homework to make me want to clean the house, work on my blog, play a board game with the kids, or give the dog a bath. As soon as I open my textbook, I am struck with an overwhelmingly urgent need to knit tiny booties for the fish, but first, I must learn to knit. Luckily, I have a book to teach me how to do this, but no needles, so I must go to the store and purchase knitting needles and a craft kit to occupy my kids so I can keep those precious fishes' tiny fins warm this winter.

OK, not really. But in the time it took me to answer ten of my math problems, I also checked my Facebook seven times, read email in two accounts, texted three people, did five jumping jacks (I swear my butt was getting larger by the minute, and I could feel imaginary blood clots forming in my legs), and started two blog entries. I also participated in my other class's discussion board, hugged the cat against his will a few times, let the dog out and in again, and drank a can of Diet Coke. I now feel a great Homework Manifesto coming on that must be written down immediately, before I forget it. I must make sure to document my objection to the word "subtended" for all of humankind. This is clearly more important than finding the area of a parallelogram. It reminds me of the little protest signs I doodled on my math folder in high school that read DOWN WITH MATH. (See, I was articulate and clever at a young age.)

Next, I poured myself a glass of wine. Note to readers: Math and wine don't mix. Wine and blogging, wine and housekeeping, wine

(continued)

and a lot of other things, OK, but wine and math, no. I no longer cared about finding the circumference of a circle, or of anything else. Although, now that I think of it, I should find the circumference of the fat rat terrier sleeping next to me. That would be fun and educational, with the added bonus of irritating the dog. But first, I should pay some bills. Paying bills is **important.** It is **necessary.** So is printing off my insurance cards and doing my taxes.

I have the perfect excuse for not doing homework—the kids are at Daddy's. My seven-year-old loves to sit on my lap and "help" me do my math. He takes his brother's toy cash register (which is also a working calculator) and calculates the numbers I give him, and recites the answer to me. It is *educational* and *bonding.* If I were to do all of my math homework without him, he might miss out on an awesome personal growth/parental bonding moment, and *that* would be bad parenting. So I paid one bill and checked Facebook two more times, and considered posting a ten-minute play I just read and loved to my writers' group. Because all of that is way more important that finding the density of a cylinder.

Here's why: Something marvelous has been invented called the internet. If, for some odd reason, I need to know the circumference of anything, I can type it into my preferred search engine and get the right answer, every time. What I can't do is use my search engine to spend quality time with the kids, clean my house, or torment the cat. Therefore, it is a simple matter of economy. I need to do what only I can do. Not math. Down with Math.

· ·

Posted by Lara L Tuesday, February 12, 2013 at 7:54 AM
Labels: Grown Up Time

THE GOOD MEN PROJECT

Home > Featured Content

What a Boy's Love of Baseball Taught His Sports-Averse Mother

I somehow always knew I'd have boys, and I was happy when I had my two. Because I assumed they would be male versions of me or maybe my brother, I was prepared to build forts, play with Transformers, and read J. R. R. Tolkien at bedtime. These were all things I liked, too. But apparently their father's genes, or his influence, or both, are stronger, because in spite of everything I have tried to do, my elder son is not the king of Legos, or chess, or swimming, or art. My child is the baseball savant.

I try to be supportive. But I was hoping for a swimmer, or a karate kid, or a Rubik's cube whiz. I would be fine building robot cats or launching a Lego toy into outer space, but I also told myself that I wouldn't push my own agenda on my kids, and would expose them to many interests and let them choose their own favorites. I just never expected baseball to be it for my older son.

He reads baseball statistics like other kids read comic books. When his Little League coach speaks, he listens raptly. Every day we devote several hours to throwing and catching and hitting and running outside, and then he throws a spongy ball into the delineated strike zone in his bedroom for another hour before bed. The kid eats, sleeps, and breathes baseball.

(continued)

I'm not saying my kid is an outstanding athlete. He's all elbows and knees. He can't ride a two-wheeler bike or even swing on a swing without me pushing him, and he's almost eight years old. Baseball is just what he does all day, every day. He plays hard and cries only when the game is canceled due to rain.

I'm glad he has passion about something, but baseball? Of all the interesting things in the world, must he pick the one thing I don't like? As I inundated both boys with art and music and science, I believed that I could shape my kids to be more like me than their sports-enthusiast father. Apparently, I was wrong about that.

Or was I? If I go back in time, I have to admit that there was a point when I too loved baseball. Back before hairspray and blue eyeshadow, back when I reigned supreme over the kickball field, when I was always one of the first picked in gym class and often team captain. When I'd chase down boys that were being stupid and hit them instead of trying to kiss them. Back when I rode my bike all day and was sweaty and didn't brush my hair. Back then, I collected baseball cards and dreamed different dreams, not caring about being proper or pretty. How did I lose that part of me along the way?

It was the last week of school my sixth-grade year, and the first time I played softball in gym class. The teacher decided to make it one pitch per batter in order to cycle through as many kids as possible; there were no balls, no strikes, no fouls. You hit it well or you were out.

I was up to bat. The teacher pitched. It was coming straight down the plate. I could visualize my bat striking that ball with a resounding THWACK! I was pretty good in gym, probably in the top 25 percent of the girls. I had nothing to fear.

I swung the bat. Not only did I miss the ball, but I comically swung around in a circle and everyone laughed. Worse still, I was the final out for my team. I was mortified, and I never recovered my gym class mojo again. By the next year I had firmly established my place as one of the last picked, where I would remain for all of junior high. I never liked team sports again.

And yet here I am, playing baseball regularly with my two boys now. After getting stung by a few fastballs, I bought myself a used mitt that I actually really like. It smells beautifully of leather and childhood. Occasionally, I am even able to catch with it, which fills me with childlike glee and a sense of accomplishment way out of proportion to what it should be. Let me tell you, in the under-eight-year-old baseball standings, I am an all-star, even though I often refuse to run for the ball.

Last week my older son and I discovered the best and biggest baseball diamond we had ever seen just a few blocks from our house, tucked away behind a church. Maybe it was the sight of the empty bleachers, or the perfectly groomed infield, but something about that place combined with the feel of the ball landing solidly in my mitt woke up a part of me that had been long dormant. I really had fun.

And I realized that mothering a baseball player has helped me regain skills that I forgot that I cared about. I brought it up with my son as we threw the ball back and forth, both of us running for grounders and pop flies.

"I think playing with you has raised my skill level to the point that I could actually play with grown-ups if I wanted to," I said as I threw the ball.

"Mama, that would be so cool. And I could give you tips and help you learn to bat if you had problems. I could totally help you get better," he said as he threw the ball back.

Kids can change you into a person you don't necessarily want to become, and that can be a good thing. Sometimes you lead, and sometimes you follow, but the more I step back and see where

(continued)

my boys are going, the more amazed I am by the journey I am taking beside them. Legos, chess, and baseball are only vehicles for talking, for healing, for teaching and for learning, and it doesn't much matter which vehicle they choose. It's the ride that matters.

But that doesn't mean I'll be signing myself up for baseball.

. . . .

Posted by Lara Lillibridge September 30, 2013
Filed Under: Featured Content, Raising Boys

Barely Recognizable Animals

I may not have had a lot of extra money, but I did have a sewing machine and a box of fabric remnants I had dragged from New York to Key West to Kansas to Ohio, and they didn't even smell funky. When Big Pants wanted a chipmunk stuffed animal, I decided to make him one instead of buying one. I could do this. I went online and found a pattern for a "pointy kitty" which I figured was similar to a chipmunk, in that it had legs, tail, and ears. I'd make the ears smaller, the legs shorter, and the tail fatter. (I actually think I got confused about squirrels and chipmunks, because chipmunk tails are not significantly fatter than cat tails.)

"I want it brown and black with a white belly," Big Pants requested. I looked through my box. I had a lot of yellow polar fleece, left over from a blanket I had never finished making. Yellow was Big Pants's favorite color, so I figured that should work.

"How about yellow?" I asked.

"OK, as long as it has a bushy tail," he said, because apparently he had also confused squirrels with chipmunks.

"One thing I can be sure of—it's going to have a bushy tail!" I answered enthusiastically. I was quite proud of myself for my resourcefulness. I was sewing away, the kids were playing nicely, and everyone was happy. Except it was becoming readily apparent that this was not going to look like a chipmunk. Or a pointy kitty. Or any kind of recognizable animal whatsoever. I gave Big Pants my button jar and distracted him with the task of choosing eyes and a nose; that way he'd be responsible for any bad stylistic decisions.

"Um, this is going to be a more imaginative animal," I said, to start letting him down slowly. I secretly praised myself for not mentioning that the back legs kind of resembled testicles. And the head resembled a creature with hydrocephalus.

"That's OK, Mama. At least it'll be yellow," he said. Yellow was the only thing I could guarantee. We didn't have any stuffing fluff, so we used scraps of fabric and cotton balls to fill the creature. I sewed on the blue button-eyes he selected, along with the shiny gold button-nose, and he was happy. He named it "Chippery" because in his four-year-old eyes it was obviously a chipmunk.

• • •

I decided that the chipmunk was such a success that I would make UnobtainiMan a bunny. I had some really soft brown fabric from a skirt that had an unfortunate dryer incident and never resembled a skirt again, and some fuzzy stuffed-animal-fur type fabric for a tail. I thought I could make an oval mini-pillow type thing and attach ears, feet, and a tail and I'd be good to go. Except the "sew it inside out and turn it right-side out" part didn't go quite according to plan and the ears wound up on top of each other, one drooping down over the face and the other sticking out like a unicorn horn. I called it Chernobyl Bunny and when he gave it a place of honor on his dresser instead of hiding it in his sock drawer, I knew it was true love.

• • •

From then on, I made the kids Barely Recognizable Animals nearly every week. Sometimes I found a free pattern online (and these generally resulted in actually recognizable animals) and other times Big Pants dragged out his favorite book—*The Encyclopedia of Animals*—and requested I make some obscure yet adorable animal. A South American bush dog. A wombat. (Did you know they have a backward-facing pouch? It's so the baby isn't covered with dirt as the mama wombat digs. Unfortunately, that also means if the baby wombat sticks his head out at the wrong time, he's likely to get shat on.) Owls, monkeys, a raccoon (it turns out that a white raccoon with a black mask looks exactly like a fox in disguise), dachshunds, cats, a badger, squirrels, rhinos, hedgehogs, a sea lion, penguins, bunnies, bunny-ninjas, and child-invented superheroes. Some of these things actually looked like the animal they were supposed to resemble, others—not so much. Most of the time their legs were different lengths and occasionally they had inexplicable camel humps. I made football uniforms for tiny store-made stuffed animals, tiny baseball gloves, bats, and hats for others. Then we graduated to Pokémon. Pokémon are incredibly easy to make, it turns out, and you can generally find a coloring book page to use as a simple pattern. If you were to look at the Pokémon I made, you might think I actually knew what I was doing.

Eventually, the boys stopped requesting stuffed animals, though I still make them things every now and then. Mainly, though, I'm trying to outsource my stuffed-animal-making to the children. For Tiny Pants's birthday, Big Pants designed and sewed a baby Ewok for his brother, complete with a detachable hood. I ran the sewing machine pedal, and he sat on my lap and guided the fabric through. It had one tiny leg and one normal one, but it was brown and fuzzy and made with love. And Tiny Pants adored it, because his big brother made it just for him.

ONLY MAMA

How We Obtained a Cat

If you are wondering what a single mama with two jobs, two kids, and one dog needs to balance her life, the answer is another pet, obviously.

Some people will caution you that:

1. Cats are a long commitment.
2. Cats will require veterinary expenditures of an unknown amount over their lifetime.
3. Cats require cat boxes that no one cleans but Mama.

However, I like cats. My boys had wanted another pet since the guinea pig had died a year previously, and I figured a cat was a hardier animal. Daddy had a dog and a cat at his house (my cat from my first marriage, to clarify) and I just had the one dog since the unfortunate demise of the guinea pig. Daddy's cat was nearing the end of her days, and the guinea pig-sized void was about to be increased by a cat-sized void in their lives.

Still, I wouldn't have done anything about it if a dear friend hadn't had a stray cat give birth to kittens in her house. The Pants brothers and I went to visit the kittens as soon as their eyes opened. The boys begged to take one home. I waffled. I was filled with fear of commitment that rivaled that of a twenty-year-old man, but they were cute, and I was the only parent, so I could get a pet if I wanted. I could get ten pets. I have to admit the freedom to buy live fluffy things was very heady, so I gave in and said *probably*, but only to one kitten. I then clarified, one kitten for the family, not one kitten each. Tiny Pants was a tad disappointed.

I bought cat food, cat litter, and a cute little dish set for the kitten I was not entirely sure I wanted to obtain. I called my vet and discussed shot schedules and costs and timing of neutering, and continued wavering. It turns out that *probably* sounds a lot like *yes* to people under four feet tall, and I already had enough Mama Guilt from the divorce, so that was that. We were getting a kitten.

Finally, the kittens were old enough to leave their mother, and with great trepidation I went sans kids to pick out a kitten. They boys had their favorites, of course, but seeing as it would be my responsibility, I figured I should get the one I really liked. I took the cutest one they had.

I brought the little guy home (yes, now my household consisted of two male children, a male dog, and a male cat) where he promptly hissed at me and hid under the furniture. Picking out an animal based on looks instead of temperament works, I tell you.

I dragged him out from under my cedar chest and placed him on the bed, where I promptly took a bunch of cute kitten pictures, at least until I noticed a flea on his leg. The vet had told me they could give him a mega flea pill if he in fact had fleas, but I had neglected to pick it up. I had fifteen minutes to get to the vet before they closed, so the kitten went into a cardboard box and I ran off to the vet, clutching the shoe box like a football. I fear flea infestation almost as much as lice infestation or death by spiders.

The kitten was given a pill and some topical stuff, and I spent the evening with him on my bed, cooing over his impossible cuteness. Well, I did for about five minutes, until slightly dead but not entirely dead fleas started dropping off him onto my white sheet. Aaaaaaaaack! There were more fleas than a two-pound animal could possibly hide on his body, and they weren't entirely dead. They were hopping. In my bed. On the bottom sheet, not on top of the comforter, because I have no foresight, apparently.

(continued)

The kitten was combed against his will and allowed to return to his hiding place under the dresser while I washed everything and vacuumed thoroughly. Said kitten was named in a less elaborate naming ceremony than I had envisioned due to the time spent in flea-de-infestation-ing.

I knew if I let the kids name him it would take days or weeks of arguing, and he'd wind up named after a football player or cartoon character, so I was claiming naming rights for myself. I would like to say I held him up to the sun, smeared ashes or crushed ocher on his forehead and said, "I Name You Grunion!" but that didn't happen. I'm not sure I even looked into his eyes and said his name with great reverence. In fact, I'm not sure I even told him that "Grunion" was a name that belonged to him, or asked his opinion of it. I just assumed he'd figure it out.

Grunion, by the way, are fish that come up on shore to breed and lay their eggs. They are an unusual fish, but not particularly attractive. Still, I loved naming a cat after a fish, and Grunion has a nice ring to it.

In a weird twist of fate, their father's cat passed away the same day I obtained the kitten surprise for them. I hadn't planned it as a transition animal but it did ease their grief, or taught them to stuff their feelings with replacement family members. Too soon to tell.

. . . .

Posted by Lara L Tuesday, February 26, 2013 at 9:34 AM
Labels: Times I Got It Right or Just Got Lucky

Budgets and Birthdays and a Complicated Cake

I was managing to provide the life I wanted for my children. As for myself, I happened upon an extremely talented hair dresser at the $9.99 hair salon down the street, and the local Goodwill had a regular donator in my exact size who had excellent taste. I stayed out of the malls, so I didn't long for what I couldn't afford. However, UnobtainiMan had slowly evolved into my most Significant Other (hereafter referred to as SigO), though we still weren't living together. He happened to have a birthday coming up, and there was no way I could buy him anything at the children's consignment store, as he was not a fan of giant sit-on ponies or train sets. Sure, I could find some random thing at Target just to have a gift, but I wanted to give him something he really loved but couldn't or wouldn't get for himself.

In conversation one day, he mentioned that his favorite cake was cassata cake, which I had never heard of. Off to Google I went, because one thing I could damn sure do was bake. I learned that it was an Italian recipe made with candied fruit, but my honey had described it as having strawberries between the layers. It took me several weeks, but I finally found a blog with the Cleveland version of cassata cake that he was referring to. Unfortunately, the five-page recipe was more complicated than anything I had ever attempted before, but the effort was the gift, so it needed to be a lot of work.

I waited until the children went to bed, then I retrieved all the measuring cups and spoons from under the couch where the baby had stashed them. I even rinsed them off, which just shows my level of commitment. I was going to make cake, pastry cream (I wasn't entirely sure what that even was), and whipped cream. Almonds were going to have to be toasted, since my grocery store didn't sell them pre-toasted, and that was something else I had to google to learn how to do. Two cakes were going to some-

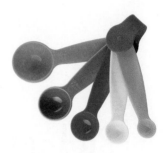

how magically get glued together. Sure, I baked in general, but this was an entirely different level of baking, particularly in my galley kitchen.

I retrieved the stand mixer (which I had won in the divorce even though it had been a gift from Daddy Pants's aunt) from the basement storage and situated it on top of the free-standing dishwasher. My heart rate was as elevated as if I were about to sing karaoke as I assembled all the ingredients, balancing them in the six inches of free space in front of the microwave. I reread the recipe, which included many threats, such as "do not over whip" and, conversely, "whisk constantly." It assumed I had weird items such as a pastry bag with star tip and cardboard rounds—items I was going to have to forgo.

I grabbed the round tin of cornstarch and added it to the pastry cream ingredients in one bowl, while whisking the heavy cream as directed. I slowly added the mixture into the cream while whisking *constantly*. It rose rapidly in a frothy, foamy cloud and overflowed down the sides of the pan. Fuck. Apparently, I had mistaken the round tin of baking powder for the round tin of cornstarch. Luckily, I had overbought on the heaving whipping cream and had enough to start over again, since a store run would have been impossible with two children sleeping upstairs. In the end, I created a five-pound plate of love and carbs and sticky goodness. And he loved me forever for it, or at least he had the good sense to say so.

Simplified Cassata Cake
(Cleveland Version)

In hindsight, a lot of effort could have been avoided with the substitution of some premade ingredients. Although it reduces "the greater the labor, the greater the gift" thing, it should save you a bunch of time.

Ingredients

Yellow cake mix, plus whatever ingredients that requires. Sometimes eggs, oil, or butter, depending. I have no idea why this isn't standard when they all taste exactly the same.

1 package vanilla pudding, which probably requires milk. Check the package before you leave the store. Someone on the internet once said that the kind of pudding you cook is far superior to the instant pudding that you just mix and go. She could be a liar who just wants you to dirty a pan, but what if she is right?

2 pints strawberries

1 package sliced almonds

1 can of Reddi Wip or possibly a tub of Cool Whip. I think Cool Whip is more delicious and airy, but I'm not sure if it will adhere to the sides of the cake or slide off. I suppose you expected me to test this for you, but I wanted you to experience the excitement of uncertainty I always feel in the kitchen.

Procedure

1. Yellow Cake. Prepare the cake according to the directions on the box, following the instructions for the 2-round-pan variety.

(continued)

2. Pudding. Again, follow the directions on the box.
3. Almond and Strawberry Preparation:
   - Chop up 1 pint of washed and de-leafed strawberries, save the other pint whole and pretty to be used as garnish.
   - Preheat oven to 350 degrees.
   - Spread nuts in one layer on ungreased shallow baking pan.
   - Bake for 10 to 15 minutes, stirring occasionally, until slightly brown and delicious smelling. You can also do this in a frying pan on the stove, but I tend to burn them less if I use the oven. I don't know why.
4. Assembly:
   - Place one cake layer onto your very best plate, or the only plate that's clean. Spread a bunch of pudding on top. Use pudding to spackle any cracks or holes in the first layer of cake because it never comes out of the pan smoothly when I do it.
   - Cover the pudding with chopped strawberries. (You may now safely eat the rest of the pudding and/or lick the bowl.)
   - Very carefully place the top layer of cake onto the strawberries. It's helpful to hold your breath and chant, "Come on, Bessie. Come on, Bessie," as you do this.
   - Cover the cake with whipped cream using a spatula, big spoon, or knife to spread as necessary. The sides are the hardest. It doesn't have to be pretty.
   - Using a flat hand, spackle the frosted sides of the cake with the almonds. Yes, your hands will become caked in both whipped cream and almonds, but then you get to lick it all off. Arrange almonds that

missed the cake and litter the plate in an artful way and pretend it was intentional.
- Top with remaining whole and chopped strawberries in a visibly pleasing manner.

Secret Benefit: My kids hate this cake so I don't have to share.

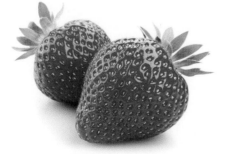

Mother F-ing Snakes on a Mother F-ing Plane, Or How I Wound Up on the Huffington Post

When I first submitted my writing various places, I had the good luck to get some acceptances by a few kind editors who were willing to work with me to shape and develop my submissions into something actually publishable. I wish I remembered their names, but that would be too much to expect of me, and if you have read this far, you already know to keep your expectations of me low when it comes to my ability to stay organized. One day SigO, formerly known as UnobtainiMan, said, "My goal for you is to get something on *Huffington Post* in the next year," and I was all, "yeah, but I'd also like a pony and I don't see that happening in the next year either, so goals are good to have but pass the Fritos," because Fritos are incredibly fantastic and there is even a place in Cleveland that sells chocolate-covered Fritos which is even more outstanding.

We used to go to a bar that had a trivia contest every week. I say "used to" because if I say I still do I'll wake up in the middle of the night paranoid that some crazed reader will look up all the trivia venues near my house and randomly show up to meet me and/or beat me at trivia. Which is ridiculous because I'm not actually all that stalk-worthy, and very few people beat me at trivia. One night we had one of those alcohol-fueled brilliant state-of-the-world-and-how-to-fix-it conversations at the bar in between trivia questions. We were both feeling jaded and negative about marriage, and were discussing how cell phone contracts are like a zillion pages long with all these terms and conditions and explanations about when and how you can sue them but marriage licenses are just a few lines on a piece of paper. The next day I wrote a slightly more coherent version and submitted it to the *Good Men Project*, a website that had been nice enough to publish me several times in the past. For once, they didn't ask me for any revisions and put it on their site right away.

I made SigO read the comments because I'm afraid of comments and was terrified of trolls. It got a fair amount of traction for a week, and then it was over and I moved on to something else.

• • •

Did you know that Facebook filters your messages? A few months later, I noticed that I had two inboxes on Facebook—my regular messages and something called "other." I was afraid *other* meant scary troll-people so I wasn't especially keen on opening it, but I had nothing else to do and SigO was working and the kids were at their father's house. Inside was a message from an Editor at *Huffington* Mother-Fucking *Post*. So of course I screamed and started shaking, but not like normal screaming where you sad "yaaay!" or "OhMyGod!" or something intelligible. Instead I just went, "Eeeeeeeeeeee!" like I was possessed by some sort of digital disconnect noti-fication. SigO noticed this and asked me why I was making repeated vowel sounds, but all I could do was point to my screen. Recently, Facebook has changed the "other" folder to "message requests" and I can no longer access that message or I would post it here so I could admire it again. I googled the editor's name with shaking hands, because I didn't want to get even more excited only to find out that it was a hoax, but lo and behold he was a real person with a real bio on *Huffington Post*.

Unfortunately, it had been about six weeks since he had messaged me, owing to that stupid mail-sorting Facebook *other mail* folder, so I was pretty sure I had missed my one chance at fame. I wrote him back anyway, and he quickly replied that he would run the piece soon and send me a link. I then spent the rest of the night inexplicably yelling, "Motherfucking snakes on the motherfucking plane!" while jumping up and down. I have never actually seen the movie *Snakes on a Plane*, but for some reason it got stuck in my head as the best expression of what I was feeling inside. A few days later my essay went live on *HuffPo* and although I should have been singing "We Are the Champions," I still kept screaming about the snakes.

Here is my first wine-induced essay on divorce, published on both the *Good Men Project* and *Huffington Post*. It came out right before my first MFA residency, where a fellow student told me, "You know *Huffington Post* isn't the same thing as being published in a real lit mag, don't you?" That was OK, though, because *Huffington* asked me to submit more pieces and eventually gave me my own permanent blog there, and last I checked she still doesn't have one.

What If We Treated Marriage More Like the Contract It Is?

I've been married twice, and both times I went into it with a lot of hope and enthusiasm. Both times, I planned to remain married to this person forever and ever, amen. And both times, I didn't. Both times, I was the instigator in the divorce.

I reflect on that often, and wonder how much we as a couple failed, and how much was a failure of the institution of marriage itself. Is marriage essentially flawed, or am I?

The word contract is used to describe both marriage and business, with one big difference; we go into marriage with a naive, "YES! Whatever, forever! Love conquers all!" Yet we enter our relationships with our cell phone companies with multipage documents. We start a relationship with our mortgage holder with at least a thirty-page document.

People sign agreements with employers committing to binding arbitration and noncompetition clauses, but we place our happiness in trust based on unspecified faith in love. I can't be the only one who thinks that maybe we need to put as much thought into the marriage contract as we do all the other contracts in our lives.

Marriage is about unspoken assumptions, and the failure of many marriages is based on people having different assumptions as

(continued)

to what constitutes appropriate behavior. There's an old adage, "Men marry women hoping that they'll never change, but women marry men hoping to change them," and in many cases I think this is true, but I don't think either view is entirely correct.

People aren't static; we change and grow, as well we should, but what about how that affects the marriage? Do we have a right to assume the person we marry will remain the person we fell in love with, even ten, twenty, thirty years down the road?

Marriage as an institution is in trouble. Half of them end in divorce. Heck, I personally have increased the divorce rate in the country by twice my fair share. I'm not purporting to be an expert on marriage, but perhaps marriage needs to change with the times.

Perhaps, when we write our vows, we need to think a little bit more about practicalities and less about abstract love. For example, it's pretty common to pledge monogamy, but how does that actually work? What constitutes cheating? Can the woman read erotica? Can the man watch porn? Is online chatting the same as cheating? What if the woman kisses a girl? How much sex does each partner expect? Under what circumstances can that change? How will each partner deal with potential changes? It seems like common sense, and I'm sure all couples talk about these nuances before marriage, but maybe writing it down would help keep everyone on the same page.

I may sound cold, but when you realize that most serious ruptures in marriages are from a failure to communicate properly, perhaps the best defense of marriage is to be a little less Pollyanna about it.

One would never sign an employment agreement that stated, "I will do whatever work the company feels is necessary, regardless of the hours or toll it takes." Yet we form households with vague divisions of labor that are often filled with animosity. No one would ever think to divide out household tasks in their marital agreements, yet that is what most people fight over. I once kicked my husband for not taking out the dog when it was his turn, then pretended I did it in my sleep and had no idea what he was talking about. Is that direct communication? No!

What would have happened if we had a clearly written document that detailed our expectations, including time spent with friends and family, managing disposable income, division of work, and raising children? What do you love best about your mate? How can you ensure that part of them doesn't change?

How will you deal with the times when compromise is necessary, and no one wants to? There was a sitcom once about two friends in business together, and each was given a set number of "insists," which they could use to dissolve an impasse. What if, in your marriage, you could say, "I'm using my insist!" when things got too heated? (This could only work if each person only had three insists a year.)

What are the "deal breakers" of your particular marriage? Mental health issues? Drug addiction? Bad behavior? Violence? Being taken for granted? Under what conditions will counseling be insisted on? What if, when you reached an intolerable point in your marriage, instead of saying, "I don't know what to do," you had already agreed on what to do?

Personally, I can't promise to live with someone "till death do us part" without some measure of "unless" involved. I don't think it's healthy to give someone a free pass to treat you however they want, or for you to treat them badly, either. I think one of the drawbacks of marriage is that it is all too easy to take our partners for granted and stop bringing our best selves to the relationship.

How might that change if you knew you had to re-sign your contract every five years, and your spouse was able to invoke the predetermined dissolution clause with pre-negotiated spousal support and division of assets? Might men and women both try a little harder to be good to one another?

(continued)

What if you got all of that fighting resolved before you spent thousands of dollars on a wedding? What would life look like if we paid as much attention to the nuts and bolts of forming a household unit as we did to the selection of the DJ for the reception?

· ·

Posted by Lara Lillibridge November 27, 2013 at 4:56 PM
Updated: January 27, 2014
More: Divorce, Contract, Wedding, Marriage Contract

PART THREE
INTO THE FAMILY BLENDER

The House Is Right, the Time Is Now

SigO and I started discussing moving in together. I loved my little single-mama house, but we were outgrowing it. I spent a lot of time fantasizing about a second toilet—even one in the basement with only a shower curtain around it like we had when I was a child. I had a couple of window air-conditioning units and had run a long extension cord into the bathroom so I could use a window fan in the summer while I did my makeup, but as soon as I walked into the hallway I was met with a furnace blast of heat, my eyeliner melted, and my hair levitated into a cloud of gravity-defying frizz. I dreamed of central air. I shared a driveway with my neighbor, and had only one covered parking spot, so if SigO moved in, one of us would have to park on the street. Adding another full-sized human to our 1,072-square-foot home was not going to work, especially since school was about to end for the summer and SigO worked from home. We started the big discussion.

He felt it was imperative that I start teaching the boys to pick up after themselves before we moved in together, so that it wouldn't look like he was the reason for the sudden rules change. I swore I was going to get right on that next week. I explained how they now had to put their dishes in the sink instead of leaving them on the table and that was a larger accomplishment than he realized. I was going to get stricter and tougher incrementally, over a few weeks . . . starting next week. Not today. Today it was always too much to handle.

We discussed parenting and living arrangements and looked for houses online, but we didn't discuss marriage. Neither one of us were interested in that. We decided instead to become "gay married." (Gay marriage wasn't legal at the time.) This meant that we drew up wills and made each other our emergency contacts at our doctors' offices. Daddy Pants and Nanny both signed as my witnesses on the Health Care Proxy that gave SigO the right to pull the plug on my life support, if it ever came to that. We wanted to be responsible, but not have to sign that paper in front of a judge and say, "till death do us part." I was not guaranteeing I would stick around unless I wanted to, by God. Besides, men stopped having sex with me once I married them, so why on earth would I want to do that again?

As soon as I signed my papers and collected all of my witnesses, I decided that I needed to leave him. It was too permanent, too real, and giving authority to someone else was just too much to bear. So I did what any sensible girl would do and I ran and fought and tried to get away, but he held me close until my demons receded and I became brave once again.

We walked thorough a couple of houses—all much larger than I was capable of cleaning, with lawns larger than I was willing to mow—and I fell in love with a brick colonial a few blocks from the beach. "If I lived here, I'd feel like a princess every day," I told him. The next day he put an offer on it, and in less than two months it was time to have all the people I loved living under one roof. This was what I had yearned for. Once our offer was accepted, though, I had to summon my courage and tell Daddy Pants.

Daddy Pants did not date. Actually, I'm sure he did date, but he had never brought a woman around the kids. The first year or two after the divorce he'd made mention of various women in passing to me, but hadn't said anything about anyone in a very long time. Now, if he were to have a woman around the kids regularly (or a male love interest for that matter) I'd google the ever-living shit out of them. I'd want their driver's license number, credit history, and internet passwords. When SigO became Officially Significant he offered to have a beer with Daddy Pants and have some sort of respectful conversation about not trying to take his place, but Daddy Pants responded with, "Why the fuck would I want to do that? And you're stupid if you let your boyfriend have drinks with your ex-husband." But he also said, "You're a good mother. I trust that you wouldn't bring someone around the kids that was a bad person." Like so many conversations with Daddy Pants, it pissed me off and touched me all at the same time.

Daddy Pants and I had a long history of mutually avoiding conflict. Our preferred method of communication was email, so we could spend hours crafting responses and/or passive-aggressively ignore entire paragraphs and reply with only a single-word answer. There was no way I was going to pick up the phone and tell him SigO and I were moving in together. It took me three days to compose the email. I hit send and waited. And waited. There was no reply. He was pissed, but he wasn't going to say so. Silence was as good as I was going to get on this subject.

A Move and a Strike

Moving day was filled with hired men and a big white truck and boxes and boxes of toys and clothes and sentimental objects. It was hot for the beginning of June, and the movers were covered in sweat and left a trail of body odor in their wake. They laughed at me as I apologized over and over for having too much stuff. They couldn't believe by how much I had crammed into my tiny house. I had six extra-large boxes of stuffed animals, plus clothes, books, toys, sporting equipment—and that was just the kids.

When I decided that the three of us would move in with SigO the boys weren't pleased. I was surprised by this, because they'd always liked him. He started spending first one night a week over at our house, then two, and eventually he'd basically moved in with us entirely. Yet, when SigO and I found this big, beautiful house with a big, beautiful yard and plenty of bathrooms and actual working fireplaces, the kids were not happy about the idea even a little bit. First of all, they liked their existing house. Unlike me, they did not mind pooping in front of family members and did not see my lust for a second bathroom as a valid reason for moving. They didn't mind the lack of central air or the tiny yard, and they resented my insistence that these things would improve our lives. Oh, they were happy to visit the new house and climb on the swing set in the backyard, but they wanted to come home to our house at night. They did not understand my insistence that

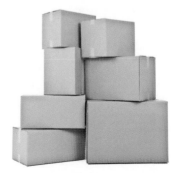

owning two houses one mile apart was impractical and expensive. They thought I was being ridiculous.

On top of that, although I'd promised to become stricter about house-keeping and chores and manners and not eating on the couch and all that stuff before we moved, I failed. SigO kept nagging me to step up my A game before the move so that the new house and the change in cleanliness expectations were unrelated. I kept promising over and over that I was going to get on that tomorrow and besides I already made them take off their shoes and carry their plates to the sink after dinner and did he not recognize what a monumental accomplishment that was? So in the end, we moved into a new house and suddenly they had all sorts of nonsensical rules about not chewing with their mouths open and not running their sticky fingers along the wall as they walked down the stairs and not eating in the living room. Oh, and once a week they had to clean their bedroom on top of it.

A week after we moved in together, the Pants brothers went on strike—without tears or even the slamming of doors. Big Pants and Tiny Pants merely exited the kitchen, walked to the driveway, got into the car, and sat there, refusing to partake in this new house thing altogether. Since it was summer I had to force them out of the car, because I was against boys baking themselves in a car-oven even though I admired their protest skills. I mean, they'd never heard of a strike or a sit-in and yet there they were, adorably organizing a show of civil disobedience. SigO wisely allowed me to break the news that we were here to stay. Since they were having such an issue with the adjustment, I had to once again email their father. Greeeeeat.

Surprisingly, Daddy Pants emerged as an ally. "They have to respect SigO," he texted back. "But they can always talk to me about their feelings. I have a stepfather, too. I understand." The tension between us dissipated, and we resumed our previous non-tense nonspeaking relationship.

Easy Like . . . Oh, Hell, Easy Is for Elevator Music

Although I had planned and dreamed of our life together for years, now that it was actually happening, it terrified me. Suddenly, I wanted to run away as fast as I could. Now that his separation had resolved itself in divorce, I had better be right about him. Now that he had moved in with my children, I needed to be absolutely sure that I wanted him to stay.

I thought that maybe I'd just keep my own place on the side for a while, vacant, until I could make sure that I was all in. My little backup plan wouldn't hurt anybody, and then if it didn't work out, it wouldn't be so hard to leave. I told him my strategy and he said, "You have to be all in." I responded, "Hell no. I want this, but I'm not ready for this all-in thing and I'll just keep paying rent for my old house. It's not bothering anyone anyway."

But he was the only one I could talk to about hemorrhoids and the fact that my rosacea had spread to my chin, giving me a sunburn goatee. Rather than laughing, he tried to help me cover it up. And he was the only one who knew about that time when I was so sad I thought I'd break apart and I crawled under the bed where the world was smaller. And he was the one I had sex with on the hood of my car in the parking lot of a building neither of us lived in, and we laughed about the tenants watching us from behind their curtains. I told myself that I was sure we could make this work and I stopped thinking about keeping a little empty house on the side like a residential mistress.

This settling into living together was harder than I thought. Every now and then, I had to make a point that I was not going to be pushed around—that I wasn't going to say *it's fine* anymore, when it wasn't fine at all. It didn't matter that he wasn't the one who pushed me around and I never said *it's fine* to him, these words had lived untamed in me throughout my previous marriages and they never got out when they should've so now they finally could—I was safe.

Doubt and fear came back in unexpected places because the children loved him too, even if they did give him back talk. That's what children do when they feel safe. God knows, they couldn't say *boo* to their father. They trusted SigO not to yell and not to leave, so they did all the age-appropriate boundary pushing with him that they didn't do at their dad's house, but it wasn't easy or joyful for any of us. For SigO, who had never had children, it was a bit like being dropped by helicopter behind enemy lines.

Once the children became too attached to him, there would be no going back. There was a big difference in my mind between divorcing while my children were still in diapers and breaking up with someone when they were six and eight years old. It didn't matter that SigO wasn't their father. I remembered how my father's multiple divorces affected me as a child—how the world seemed unstable and as if nothing were ever permanent. I had thought that I was so sure about this step, but I had lived six years alone without anyone second-guessing my parenting, cleaning schedule, or budget. Freedom was hard to give up, no matter how badly I wanted a new life. I have never been good at compromise.

Every time we argued over our blended lives—how to raise the children or how much interaction he should have with his ex-wife—I ran to my children's bedroom on the third floor. If the boys were at their father's, I buried myself in Big Pants's bed, my head on his ladybug pillow. I breathed in his scent and clutched one of his stuffed animals to my chest. When the boys were home, I curled myself around Tiny Pants's sleeping body and pretended that he didn't know I was there. We had bought their new beds just for this room, just for this house. I knew the cheap particleboard frames were not strong enough to survive a move, and the children weren't, either. Whenever I thought that we must leave and start over again it was these beds—chosen so carefully and foolishly, dragged up three flights of stairs and assembled with many curse words—that made me cry. They could never be disassembled and reassembled and remain salvageable. And SigO always came upstairs and led me back to our bed, where we both knew I belonged, leaving both the boys and their beds safe once more.

• • •

SigO didn't yell at the kids or reprimand them once for probably the entire first year. Instead he'd wait for them to go to bed and then discuss ~~his demand list~~ parenting strategy with me, and I'd get to be the bearer of bad news. We fought about children and rules and bedtime and I compromised, and I remembered that I left the children's father because I refused to compromise, and I worried that there was something very wrong with this. But I knew that this time, I was parenting with someone who spent a lot of time thinking about how to raise children so they became successful adults and not overindulged brats, and I knew he wasn't just trying to be selfish. SigO had been dropped into active parenting duty with no training and little warning. He hadn't had the benefit of having first one baby, then two, who grew slowly into stubborn little people. Rather, he was trying to figure out his place with two children who had reached the age of sass. I knew that I let those children walk all over me and I knew they needed to be reined in by someone. I trusted him to be gentle about it, but I still made sure it was my voice telling those urchins I mean darlings to put their toys away and their dishes in the sink, because it needed to be my voice, not his, at least most of the time that first year. When the kids crowded my thoughts and face and there was no breathing room, it felt good to lean back and rest on his chest, strong and safe. His arms came around me and he made sure those children I mean demons didn't overwhelm me. He'd make sure that neither the children nor my demons overwhelmed me.

• • •

At night we laughed by the fire and had a glass of wine or three, and I thought that everything was fine in the world, and it was, until the next time that life's aggravations cropped up and it all became a lot more work than they told me it would be in fairy tales. He loved that I was goofy and talked too much, and that I danced silly dances in the kitchen and sang off-key throughout the house. All I could think was that I hoped that he never tired of my goofy dances in the kitchen and that he always loved my lopsided smile. Let's be honest, he really didn't love my off-key singing, but he said that he did and I told him that he had better because I was not going to stop off-key singing—I couldn't. I was too happy. Although I secretly worried that he would tire of me, at least this uncertainty meant that I was crazy in love and not indifferent. I was glad and grateful that I had found him even if our life together wasn't always wrapped up with a pretty ribbon. Fairytales were dull anyway. And when I told him that I had written an essay, he replied with, "Yo, *esé*!" with a Spanish accent. I did my best impression back, and then he made me read it aloud even though it was one in the morning, and afterward we fell into bed together laughing.

• • •

Last summer, a friend told me, "You make sense together. It's like you are the male and female mirror of each other." Sometimes relationships start under the worst of circumstances, but sometimes messy inappropriate beginnings lead to the right ending.

ONLY MAMA

HOME | POSTS | ABOUT THIS BLOG | ABOUT ME

The Best Advice I Have Ever Been Given

A few nights ago, I was very upset and stewing into the early morning hours over a fight I had with a loved one. I was quite sure that I was entirely right and they were entirely wrong. I asked on Facebook if anyone else was up—it was four o'clock in the morning—and an online writer friend I've never met in real life replied. She lives in Guernsey (an island in the English Channel) where it was a perfectly normal time to be awake.

I typed out my anger and heartbreak, and she said:

Listen to me very carefully, because I have to go pick someone up at the airport in five minutes.

OK, I typed, my heart full of hope for the One Great Answer that would change my life. She was a single mama, too. I was sure that her struggles led to Deep Insight, I was confident that her next words would change my life.

Go to sleep. It's the middle of the night. You aren't going to resolve anything at four o'clock in the morning.

That was it. No judgment, no commiserating, no comment on my Great Personal Struggle.

Go. The F*ck. To Sleep. (I added the obscenity; she's far too polite for that.)

She was right. Sleep didn't magically fix anything, but it certainly was better than mentally picking at sores all night and resolving nothing.

(continued)

It's 4:00 a.m. There are no magic words. Go to sleep and try and become rational.

Had another friend answered, we might have stayed up for the rest of the night rehashing all my feelings and arguments and doing nothing but making me more sleep deprived. Instead, she Mama'ed me and put me to bed.

Go to sleep. It will be better in the morning, or at least the same in the morning, but you'll be less tired at least. It is truly the best advice we can give anyone in the middle of the night.

Thanks, Limpet Girl.

. . . .

Posted by Lara L Wednesday, July 2, 2014
Labels: Advice, Friends, Not My Finer Moments, Single Parenting, Sleep

Instant Oatmeal Cookies

If you have recently entered the family blender you deserve a treat. However, if you put off buying groceries and have nothing in your cabinets that resembles a treat, it is helpful to know how to make cookies out of random things when you are stressed out and are having a cookie emergency and have no freaking ingredients for cookies in the house, which happens to me quite often.

The end result is more cookie-esque than cookie, but it is tasty and requires a minimum of supplies.

Ingredients
¼ cup sugar (I suspect that if you use plain oatmeal you may need more sugar)
2 packets instant oatmeal, any flavor. I used maple because I buy a box of assorted flavors of oatmeal and I don't like maple-flavored oatmeal, so I always have plenty left over. It's gross for breakfast, but it makes a fine cookie.
5 teaspoons melted butter

Procedure
1. Cover cookie sheet in tinfoil. Do not use nonstick spray or anything fancy like that.

(continued)

2. Mix sugar and oatmeal together. Note: you can also add nuts and raisins. Probably chocolate chips if you have them, but I didn't. I did have something left over from a salad that looked like nuts and were called "pepitas" so I threw them in, because I like nuts and seeds, even ones I have never heard of.

3. Add butter slowly, in case you have too much or too little butter, depending on how much overflowed in the microwave when you were melting it. You don't want soup.

4. Spoon onto pan. It won't look anything cookie-like. It's kind of like you pour the stuff on the cookie sheet, then you form it into lumps that are vaguely cookie-shaped. I made 6 cookies, but you could probably make more or fewer depending on the size of cookie you like and the size of the pan you have.

5. Bake 10-ish minutes on 350. The bigger the cookie, the longer the bake time. As always, turn on the oven light and look through the window. Sadly, my oven light was out, so I had to open and peek. This is actually not that bad, because it releases clouds of cookie fragrance.

6. Let cool until firm, and kind of smush them together a little as they cool. Of course, if you really need a cookie this minute and can't wait for them to firm up, just eat them with a fork.

Sleepover with Daddy Pants

The Cleveland Air Show happens every Labor Day, and every year, SigO gets free tickets. We invited Big Pants's best friend to spend the night Friday, since Daddy Pants had relatives coming on Saturday and was taking the boys a day early. I try to always schedule sleepovers so that the boys go to Daddy's house the following day when they are overtired and cranky. However, that morning, Tiny Pants came downstairs and informed me that Big Pants was unable to walk. He'd been having pain in his hip since we went to a water park a few days earlier, but it had gotten so bad that he could no longer walk down the stairs, or even crawl. I piggybacked him to the living room and carefully deposited him on the sofa. I called the doctor, who offered that I could pick up some crutches and see if the issue would resolve itself on its own, or I could take him to the ER for diagnostics. Not being a huge fan of vague undiagnosed illnesses nor of carrying my nine-year-old up and down the stairs, I thought we'd run down to the local hospital and get a quick X-ray before his best friend came over to spend the night. I brought Tiny Pants along (SigO was in Florida, where I was supposed to join him on Saturday) but I neglected to bring any snacks, books, or toys, since I had called ahead and been assured that the hospital wasn't busy. Forty-five minutes, tops, I advised the best friend's father.

Except they didn't have a pediatrician available to read the X-ray. So we sat. I installed a video game on my cell phone to entertain the kids—something I swore I would never do. I fed the family out of the vending machine. I started reciting *The Hobbit* by J. R. R. Tolkien from memory. Around dinnertime—seven hours after we arrived—Daddy Pants arrived and the doctor told us that Big Pants had fluid in his hip and needed to go to the Cleveland Clinic downtown. No sleepover party. No air show. And he had to transfer hospitals by ambulance.

Apparently, there are parents who refuse medical treatment for their children and/or flake out if the treatment seems too inconvenient, so they wouldn't allow me to drive him thirteen miles to the main campus by myself. "Of all the parents we get in here, I am quite confident that you of all people would actually show up with him downtown," the nurse confided to me, "but they won't allow me to release him into your custody."

The real problem with the ambulance ride was that only one person could accompany him, and Daddy Pants and I each had our own cars there.

"Who do you want to ride with you?" I asked Big Pants. "It doesn't matter. Neither of our feelings will be hurt. It's totally up to you." I felt terrible asking him to choose between his parents, but I didn't know what else to do.

"It doesn't matter," he said.

"Are you sure?" I asked.

"Completely."

"I'll ride with him," Daddy Pants said. That thing about it not mattering who rode in the ambulance? Turns out, I lied. It mattered to me quite a lot.

Daddy Pants had kept custody of our yellow lab, who was now an elderly dog that had to go outside frequently. I had kept custody of our rat terrier, who was the same age but, in the way of small dogs, less elderly. Besides, Asterisk knew where to find my extra key and had already picked him up and brought him to her house. We decided that Daddy needed his car more than I did in order to let the dog out, so I left mine in the hospital parking lot (which was near my house) and drove his car downtown while he rode in the ambulance. Do you see how it would have been easier if I had ridden in the ambulance? Not that I'm bitter or anything. At least Tiny Pants rode with me.

First of all, if you ever have to take your child to the hospital, Cleveland Clinic is the place to go. They not only had a play area for patients and siblings, but also an Xbox and games that can be checked out and brought to your room on a cart. There was a McDonald's in the building—one of the few places my kids would reliably eat. If you've seen all those fundraisers and commercials for the Ronald McDonald House and wondered how great it could possibly be seeing as it was run or owned by a fast-food chain, I'm here to tell you that it's actually pretty great. They had a suite for parents complete with recliners that tilted all the way back into beds, showers, toiletries, and snacks—not that we used any of it. Both Daddy Pants and I refused to leave Big Pants's side. Which became a problem.

The hospital room had one bed, which was occupied by Big Pants, his IV, and his bad leg. There was one hard-backed chair, and one foldout loveseat. There was no way in hell that I was going to share a bed with Daddy Pants, and the feeling was mutual. I tried to encourage Tiny Pants to go home with Asterisk, but he refused. We were a family, and we were going to stay as a family and all sleep in the hospital room.

Daddy called the first turn of sleeping on the foldout bed. He snuggled up with Tiny Pants and they both fell promptly asleep. I walked down to the lovely Ronald McDonald House suite where a few other parents were sleeping, but under no circumstances did I want to be that far away from my kid. I needed to be able to watch the rise and fall of his chest as he slept. I went back to the room and pulled the hard-backed chair up to the foot of the hospital bed, and lay half on the chair, and half on the bed.

I knew how to sleep in hospitals. My first husband nearly severed his leg in a motorcycle crash, and I spent weeks sleeping beside him in a recliner chair. First, you adjust the hooks of your bra to the loosest setting, and loosen the shoulder straps as well—but don't take it off. The nurses are in and out all night, and doctors make their rounds around 5:00 a.m. Take off your glasses, but keep them in your pocket for the same reason. What I was no longer used to doing was sleeping to the sound of my ex-husband's snoring. It had been six years since I'd heard it last, but my body remembered as if it were the sound of my high school alarm clock, or the refrain of a detested pop song stuck on repeat. There should be a word for nostalgia with a serrated edge.

But one thing I've learned through my single-mama years is that if I'm tired enough, I can sleep anywhere, and even a few hours is enough to function. Soon enough, I managed to do just that.

The next morning Big Pants was scheduled for his MRI, and again, only one parent could accompany him. This time I didn't defer to anyone. "I'm going," I said. The nurses gave him a new toy, donated by some kind people. He held it for a moment, and asked them to save it for another kid who needed it more. His body looked so small as they slid him into the machine.

I sat at the open end by the top of his head, where he could hear me. My necklace floated in the air, attracted to the magnets. When he started to freak out in the close confines of the tube—something adults do, too—I once again recited *The Hobbit*, and spoke to him of dwarves, goblins, elves, and a dragon named Smaug. His breathing calmed. I skipped over the part when Thorin Oakenshield was slain in battle.

Let me say right here that if at all possible, it's best to avoid going to the hospital on Labor Day Weekend. There was no one available to read the MRI, so Big Pants, Tiny Pants, Daddy Pants, and I had to stay another night at the hospital. Daddy Pants's aunt was in town for the holiday, so she watched his dog, and when she came to the hospital to visit I availed myself of the opportunity to retrieve my car from the other hospital's parking lot and go home to change.

"I took the bed the first night because I figured we wouldn't be here a second night," Daddy Pants confessed when I told him smugly that it was my turn for the sofa. In that moment, I felt no regret over divorcing him. None whatsoever. Tiny Pants and I took the pull-out, and Daddy Pants scooted Big Pants over and shared the hospital bed with him.

"It's a lot more comfortable than the pull-out," he told me the next morning.

The doctor discussed aspirating the fluid in Big Pants's hip, and Daddy Pants and I both agreed that we would only allow it if they sedated him first. I'd had a procedure on my knee when I was twelve, and I still remembered the pain. We might not have been ideal roommates, but we were both on the same page when it came to the kids.

Luckily, the fluid dissipated enough on its own that Big Pants was released the following day with a pair of crutches that Tiny Pants was incredibly jealous of. The Pants brothers went to Daddy's for the rest of the weekend as planned, and I caught the last plane out to Key West to join SigO that evening.

ONLY MAMA

HOME | POSTS | ABOUT THIS BLOG | ABOUT ME

In Which We Take Dog to the Vet

If you read my post about Dog's allegedly fragile self-esteem, you know Dog has been acting out lately. He's particularly fond of shredding grocery bags, both disposable and reusable. I was concerned about this sudden obsession, so we took him to the vet.

I did some googling about suddenly destructive dogs, and I was worried about toothaches and brain tumors, so I figured before I yelled at Dog excessively I should rule out any medical problems.

ME: Dog has never been destructive. Now every morning I wake up to a pile of shredded things.
VET: Well, he doesn't have a tumor. He's walking fine, there's no indication of neurological issues. His teeth are fine. No fever. He looks happy.
ME: He's eleven now, and my ex has a dog that is also eleven and that can no longer go all night without going to the bathroom. Maybe he's frustrated that he has to hold it too long?
VET: Wouldn't he just go on the floor instead of shredding things? (Looks at me like I am a nutcase who knows nothing about dogs.)
ME: Well, there's a lot of construction near our house. Could he be stressed out from all the noise?
VET: Wouldn't he shred stuff during the day, then? Why would he wait to shred stuff at night when it was quiet?

(continued)

(I was starting to think he thought I was an idiot. I was starting to think he had a point.)

VET: He could've developed obsessive-compulsive disorder. We could give him Prozac. Are you sure he has never been destructive before? It's rare for a dog to suddenly develop destructive tendencies.

ME: No, he's never been destructive. (*awkward pause*) Well, he used to eat crayons, action figures, blocks, and Thomas trains. But nothing that was mine.

(Um, wait. Dog has always been destructive. He just ate the kids' stuff. I never cared until it was my stuff. Yes, I did just pay someone $47 to have the realization that I may be selfish and self-centered. Just a bit.)

VET: And when did he stop eating all the plastic toys?

ME: When I made the kids clean the house regularly.

VET: So he's always been destructive and ate plastic.

ME: Well, yes.

VET: Have you considered buying him a chew toy?

ME: Um, no.

VET: They sell them at many stores. Dogs like them.

MORAL #1 = Keeping a clean house is stressful to Dog.

MORAL #2 = I am an asshat who only cares when the dog eats my stuff.

MORAL #3 = Dog is just an asshat.

. . . .

Posted by Lara L Sunday, October 26, 2014 at 12:22 PM

Labels: Not My Finer Moments, Parenting, Pets

Watching Your Child Mourn

It started with a Facebook message I received at 5:30 a.m. informing me that one of Big Pants's classmates had died of complications of asthma. He was the first person my boys knew personally who died. Not just that—Collin was a boy that we all really liked, even though he lived too far away for many playdates. I always wished he lived closer. That morning, I pulled my nine-year-old son onto my lap and told him that Collin had died. Big Pants cried. I cried. Tiny Pants cried. I knew from the Facebook mom that the school was going to make an announcement in class. I thought it might help Big Pants to be with his friends, so I took both boys to school, and I went to the fourth-grade classroom with Big Pants.

• • •

The teachers had tears running down their cheeks as they told the students what happened. Many of the children wept, and I dutifully handed out tissues. One of my sons' closest friends curled his body over his desk, folding a paper over and over in his hands and not looking at anyone. Two boys squeezed into a small chair together and just sat there, not speaking.

I saw teachers crying in the halls while watching their students for clues as to how they could help—a hug, a tissue, a chance to run around or sit by themselves. I realized teachers spend more time each day with these kids than practically anyone else, certainly more than most relatives. I saw the whole school's staff try their hardest to pull themselves together for their students. They canceled classes for all of fourth grade, and we picked up Tiny Pants from his classroom and we all went home.

We didn't know what to do with ourselves at home, either, so we went to the movies. Daddy Pants came to the theater after the movie got out and hugged both the boys.

. . .

That night at bedtime, Big Pants said, "Mama, I don't know how to close my eyes to go to sleep. Every time I try I just cry and cry." All I could do was hold him, offer him books, turn on an audiobook. Eventually, he fell asleep. There were no classes the next day, either, and then it was the weekend.

I had already bought tickets to take the boys on our annual trip to see Santa downtown. We take the Unnecessary Train—we could drive there faster, but trains are fun—we watch the Christmas show, and we do our holiday shopping. The Santa bit is a twenty-minute experience in a magical workshop filled with colorful elves. Although it felt like the world had ended, Santa was the best I had to offer, so we got on the train as scheduled.

Big Pants cried driving to the train. He cried during the slow part of the Christmas show. He cried waiting to see Santa. I picked up my child who was too big for my lap and held him as he cried. Walking in the mall, it occurred to Big Pants that Collin would never get to see Santa again. He sat down on the floor right there and sobbed. I sat down on the floor next to him in the middle of the mall and held him. I started to tell him, *don't cry, it's OK,* but I corrected myself. "You can cry. Nothing about this is OK," I told him instead.

I'm sure the other parents waiting to see Santa wondered if my child had an emotional disorder or dreaded disease. Thankfully, no one asked. I could not have answered without crying myself. I thought about the Christmas presents Collin's parents must have already bought their son, hidden away in a closet or attic somewhere, that now would never be opened. I told myself I was not going to cry in Santa's Workshop, but it wasn't an easy promise to keep.

. . .

When we went in to see Santa (and we are all still Believers) Big Pants couldn't speak to Santa at all—the tears were too close to the surface. Big

Pants was only a millimeter more on the not-crying than crying scale, just enough to keep the tears from spilling down his cheeks. When Santa asked him what he wanted, he couldn't come up with a single word and just shrugged. I reminded him of his list: *a hat with a pompom, slippers to leave at school.* He just shook his head. None of it mattered to him anymore.

God Bless that Santa for understanding.

"Do you like surprises?" he asked, and elicited a nod.

"Then you'll be excited to come downstairs and see a mountain of socks and underwear under the tree?" Santa asked. My son laughed a real laugh, and the photographer caught it just inside the frame, but barely.

•   •   •

I ordered the one picture that had a smile from the Santa-Picture-Pushers even though the grouping was off-center and Big Pants was sliding off Santa's lap. That picture was my miracle.

•   •   •

When I got home, though, I didn't bother taking the picture out of the envelope. The picture I bought was a lie—a souvenir of a happy day that never existed. It was one of those moments you can look back on in years to come when you want to remember only the happy times, but that's not who we were that day. We were so sad that we left our house an hour early because we couldn't stand the feel of motionless time and grief.

•   •   •

We watched *A Charlie Brown Christmas* and that seemed to help. The sort of depressing cartoon helped him to feel not so alone. "I'm sad, too, Mama, even though it's Christmas," Big Pants said. Tiny Pants told us a story about a horse named Buttocks and I heard real laughter for a moment. I knew Big Pants would alternate being okay with not being okay for a long time. I kept that Santa picture to remind myself when I lose hope of my child ever being OK again that there's a smile waiting just around the corner. Maybe that's Santa's Christmas gift to me.

The Great Latke Incident of 2014

Life moves on, even when it feels as if it shouldn't. Big Pants's class was having a multicultural celebration party instead of a Christmas party, pre-arranged long before Collin died. A multicultural celebration probably sounded like a reasonable idea to someone who probably had a strong sense of cultural identity and who also had a tradition of delicious regional food lovingly prepared by their family. I had neither. Daddy Pants is Irish and German, but I was not going to spend a day in the kitchen paying homage to his family in spite of my own culinary failings.

My father is English all the way back to the Revolutionary War. The only things my father ever cooked were lemon chicken, assorted fishes with lemon, liver with the tears of small children, and soft-boiled eggs, none of which I was going to force upon a room of sweet nine-year-olds. My mother is half-English (which we'll ignore, as their culinary delights were covered in the sentence above) and half Russian-Jewish, which I planned to exploit for the party. Although I craftily managed to manipulate my innocent child into choosing Israel for his country (hey, it's the only foreign country where we still have living relatives), I was left with one problem: my mother had not provided me with a rich ethnic culinary history. In fact, as soon as my parents obtained a microwave oven, she stopped cooking altogether. The family just lined up in front of the microwave at night and everyone nuked their own meal. (My favorite were these premade cheeseburgers which I ate with no condiments whatsoever.) My mother did try at the occasional

Passover Seder to force me to eat gefilte fish, but I successfully resisted that sad tuna-looking thing that came in a pickle jar and was presented on a limp and soggy piece of iceberg lettuce. I knew it must be ghastly because it was the only food item I have ever successfully resisted eating—my mother had a one-bite rule for everything else. I recall her making latkes once and only once, but since no one in the family ate them she never made them again. In fact, the only traditional Jewish food I have any fond memories of was matzo, but I wasn't enough of a slacker to send my son to school with only a box of crackers.

The other problem with this cultural diversity class party was that I forgot about it until a week before it was due, and then our entire family got the flu, and Big Pants missed school for an extra week. We were all grieving and coughing and just trying to make it until bedtime. It made it hard to focus on homework. Before I knew it, it was the day before the party and we were still expected to have something to turn in. Several somethings, actually. A flag, a banner, and an ornament representing our country, all with well-researched facts, plus a dish to share with everyone. Big Pants is a huge proponent of honesty and fairness, so he insisted on making a flag for both Palestine and Israel, and copied the country names in Arabic and Hebrew. I knew that there was no way we could make latkes for twenty as well. Because I'm only half-Jewish, I Facebook messaged a couple of fully Jewish friends and asked them if there was a frozen latke or perhaps hash brown that I could pass off as homemade. They denied the existence of such a lifesaving cheat. We were going to have to do this thing the proper way, relying on Google for instruction.

Big Pants was totally happy to peel potatoes (yay!) but when I tried to show him how to grate using the new grater I had purchased just for this occasion, all we got was a handful of mush. I was about to collapse into a pool of despair when SigO walked in, foolishly thinking he could refill his

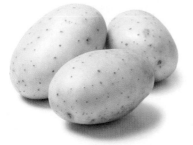

coffee cup and return to the living room. Now I may not have always made the best choices in my long-term relationships, but one thing I have done consistently is dated men who can cook. I cannot underscore the importance of this enough, particularly if you are me and kind of suck at domesticity.

SigO, God love him, actually knew how to grate potatoes. He and Big Pants grated the potatoes and chopped the onion together quite happily. All I had to do was fry them. And yes, I did sing "I bring home the latkes, fry 'em up in the pan . . ." because I'm incredibly original in my songwriting abilities. The only remaining problem was that I had not seen a real latke in thirty years and had no idea what they were supposed to look like. Again, thank you Google for helping me fake my way through parenthood.

"Mama! They look just like the picture on the internet!" Big Pants proudly proclaimed, looking over my shoulder.

I had always thought the whole food-is-love thing was about feeding people you loved. I had no idea that cooking together was a form of love, too. And that year, our mourning, still slightly feverish family found laughter and peace for an hour in the kitchen. We needed that more than we needed latkes, which I learned afterward could, in fact, be purchased frozen at Trader Joe's.

How to Make Latkes

Ingredients
1 pound potatoes
1 small onion
1 egg, beaten
½ teaspoon salt
Olive oil

Procedure
1. Wash, peel, and grate a pound of potatoes, putting the grated strips into a bowl of cold water. Let sit in cold water for ten minutes. I have no idea why, but apparently this is essential as all the internet recipes agree on this ostensibly useless step. If you are like me and are easily overwhelmed in the produce section and need the most specific of instructions, buy baking potatoes.
2. Chop up one small onion. (I used a yellow one. No clue if this matters or not, but it looked like the right size.)
3. Pour potatoes into strainer, then place with onions in a *clean* dishtowel. Roll up into a towel-burrito to remove excess water. Why you add them to water and then remove it is still a mystery to me, but I trust this is necessary.
4. Shake potato gratings and onion out of towel and into bowl. Stir in one beaten egg and ½ teaspoon of salt. Mix with hands because that adds love. I suppose a spoon also works if you aren't feeling particularly loving that day. No judgment.
5. Pour about a half inch to an inch of olive oil into a frying pan and heat up (medium-high, you don't want the

(continued)

oil to smoke because that is stinky and also somewhat scary, trust me on this). Spoon clumps about the size of a small fist of potato/onion/egg goo into the hot oil. Try to lower somewhat carefully so you don't splatter hot oil on your hands. Form into a vague hamburger patty shape with spoon and fork while they cook. Try not to touch them too much or they will fall apart. Turn heat down to medium-low-ish so you don't burn off your arm hair. Cook about five minutes, then flip over and cook five minutes on the other side. They should be no browner than a paper bag—not as light as a golden retriever and not as dark as Hershey's chocolate.

6. Cool on a paper-towel-lined plate to soak up some of the oil. You can salt more if you like salt, but I don't so I didn't.

7. Serve with applesauce or sour cream. (If you are sending them to a fourth-grade class, skip the sour cream because it'll spoil by afternoon and the kids won't eat it anyway.)

Magical Thinking

During these weeks following Collin's death, Tiny Pants had been unusually quiet. I thought, hopefully, that he was just young enough not to have been equally decimated by grief. Then one evening Tiny Pants and I were sitting at the computer, which was placed on an antique flip-top desk. He pushed his hands down on the folding desktop—something he knows he is not supposed to do—and I said something like, "Do you know how mad Mama would be if you break this desk?"

"You would never forgive me," he answered.

"There is nothing you could ever do that Mama would never forgive. Never." I replied. I was glad of this conversation, because I wanted him to always remember that he can depend on my love, even when he's a teenager, even when he does bad things. It often seems that of my two children, Tiny might be more likely to cause some major havoc someday.

"There's somebody I will never forgive," he answered. I still didn't realize that the conversation was bigger than just about breaking rules and unconditional love.

"Who?" I asked, still thinking about what a good job I was doing talking about love and forgiveness.

"Asthma."

And then I realized I wasn't doing that good of a job at all. I forgot that the two-and-half-year age gap between my sons left my youngest vulnerable. I had focused primarily on the loss his older brother had experienced. Tiny Pants may not have known this child as well, but he was still wrecked by grief.

"I know, honey," I said, and hugged him. I thought it was over. It wasn't.

Big Pants had fallen and bruised his knee earlier that day and was, in my opinion, milking it to avoid doing homework and going to bed on time. I made some comment about how if he kept having problems with his joints we'd have to go back to the hospital for some tests. This was partially a scare tactic (and a bad one) to get him to go to bed, but also voiced some real concern. After his hospital visit the doctor had said that continued joint pain might be a sign of rheumatoid arthritis, and I was just enough of a hypochondriac to worry.

At bedtime Tiny Pants started to cry. "I don't want Big Pants to go to the hospital again," he said.

At that moment I knew that this little boy's head was full of fear and death and mourning, even though he acted fine during the day and only complained about things like putting his plate in the dishwasher. Our not talking about his grief and fear had not made them go away.

Sometimes all we can do is hold our children when they cry. Sometimes we utter reassurances that we know we can't sustain, but we have to say something. That week, I was reminded that acting normal doesn't mean that grief has passed. My hope that he had magically healed hadn't made it so. The only helpful thing I knew about grief is that although it doesn't go away over time—consistently reappearing in unexpected moments—it does gradually lessen on a day-to-day basis. And it slowly ebbed from my children's lives.

Collin's parents asked in lieu of flowers to give a Christmas ornament that reminded us of their son. I picked out a hand-blown glass ornament of a wolf, Collin's favorite animal. I bought two identical ones. OK, I hadn't meant to buy two, but the flu and the grief and the online shopping "buy now" button conspired to give me exactly what we needed: I sent one ornament to Collin's parents and kept one for ourselves. Every year Big Pants hangs the wolf on our tree, and is quiet for a moment. Then he selects another ornament, and moves on.

ONLY MAMA

HOME | POSTS | ABOUT THIS BLOG | ABOUT ME

The Talk and "The Book"

I recently bought a set of three sex education books and gave the boys the first two of the set. The first was called *It's Not the Stork* for ages four and up, and its companion, for older children, was called *It's So Amazing*. I had botched any attempt at having an appropriate discussion about babies the last few times the boys had asked—I fumbled around with words about the difference between origin stories in religion versus science, and added something about magic goo. They stopped asking me anything about how babies were made altogether, and it occurred to me that they might assume that I didn't even know myself. I realized I was about to lose control over the flow of information—if they decided Mama was an unreliable source of truth, they would start asking other people instead. I figured a couple good books were the way to go.

I let the boys discover the books on their own, and when they did, I told them they could read them alone or we could read them together, or they could not read them at all. Big Pants voted to read the books on his own. I tucked the boys into bed that night, and Big Pants fell asleep reading one of the books. By some miracle, it migrated to his younger brother's bed by morning.

I waited for the questions to start, but none were forthcoming. I wondered if I should bring it up or not, but decided to wait a little longer. Finally, at dinnertime, Tiny Pants had something to say.

(continued)

"Well, that book answered one question I've had for a long time," Tiny Pants said.

"What was that?" I asked.

"How girls pee. It's called *the opening of the Virginia*."

"Actually, babies come out of their mamas' bodies through the vagina, but they pee through their urethra," I clarified.

"No, it's called the *opening of the Virginia*."

"Vagina," I insisted, abandoning the urethra discussion altogether and focusing on his pronunciation.

"Virginia."

I gave up.

A few days later we flew to Florida for a family vacation. Tiny Pants brought The Book. We were seated in the back of a full flight, elbow-to-elbow with strangers, though luckily, Tiny Pants had a window seat, so he was between me and the wall. He pulled out The Book.

"Mama, is it pronounced *Ah-Noos*?" he asked.

"No, it is Ay-Nus."

"Is it *Vel-vah*?"

(Oh God, please don't let the people around us be listening. I know that's a poorly constructed sentence, but I can't think clearly.)

"No, it is VUL-VAH," I explained. I was trying really hard. Really, I was. I wished he would ask Daddy instead. I wished for that as hard as I could.

After vacation, The Book accidentally went to Daddy's house. I was hoping it would stay there and Daddy could deal with it. No such luck. It reappeared the following week in the Daddy-And-Mommy-Bag we use to transfer toys between houses.

At this point, Big Pants had finished reading both of the books I had given him—the one for ages four and up and the one for ages seven and up. Tiny Pants really wanted his brother to read *It's Perfectly Normal,* the book for ages ten and up, even though Big Pants is only nine. I thought about it. He was almost nine and a half. He was close.

"Big Pants, do you want to read the last book?" I asked.

"Oh, Mama, I have enough knowledge for now. I'll wait for September," he replied.

Tiny Pants became frustrated with his own reading ability, so he asked me to read The Book to him. Every night I read just a few pages. We went through the names of all of the body parts, inside and out, for both sexes. We even discussed circumcision. Then one night I saw that the next night we would be reading the Penis goes in the Vagina part. Oh Lord, give me strength. I was not ready for this.

Miraculously, Tiny Pants lost interest. The next night, he requested I read *Diary of a Wimpy Kid* instead of The Book. The same thing happened the next few nights. My mother used to say that "God watches out for fools and drunks," but apparently Someone has their eye on really uncomfortable mothers as well.

Eventually I had to tell the children the basic penis-into-the-vagina mechanics. I heard that Big Pants was due for The Talk at school during health class, and I had to make sure that he knew the score. I remember being mortified in fifth grade when we had the big sex talk at school and I didn't know what fallopian tubes were. How had my mother neglected to teach me about the alien arms of the uterus?

I sat the boys at the kitchen table and briefly and quickly said something rapid fire like, "the-penis-goes-into-the-vagina-and-

(continued)

transfers-sperm-do-you-have-any-questions?" And I added something about doctors being able to accomplish the same in same-sex relationships or if people had medical difficulties conceiving, because we have friends in both camps, and I am nothing if not inclusive.

Big Pants just wanted to get away from that table faster than I did, but Tiny Pants had a few questions:

"Did you need a doctor to get pregnant with me?" he asked.

"No. Anything else?"

"When a woman has her period, does she wrap her entire body in toilet paper like a mummy?"

"Umm, no. They make special pads for that." (Tampons were not a discussion I was ready to have, nor was I going into menstrual cups. But seriously—how often did he see mummified women walking down the street?)

. . . .

Posted by Lara L Monday, March 16, 2015 at 9:43 AM
Labels: Not My Finer Moments, Parenting, Sex Talks

How to Fly
with Small Children

Flying is different than driving. Your children are not locked up in car seats, there are other people who can be irritated by your children very easily, and you can't bring everything you own. It's manageable, though, with a little preparation, even if you don't own a DS handheld electronic gaming device thingy.

As a child, my brother and I flew from New York to Alaska a few times a year, starting when I was four. By the time I was ten or eleven we flew "unaccompanied minor" with flight attendants helping us change planes, and by thirteen I did it totally on my own, navigating airports and boredom with alacrity. I know a lot about being a kid on an airplane.

I started taking my own kids on airplanes by myself when they were nine months old and three years, respectively, and have done so at least once a year since. We are travel pros, and I am always complimented on their awesome plane behavior by random strangers. I am also secretly proud that we fly often but their father only flew with them once since the divorce and had to enlist his sister as backup. Tiny Pants threw up all over him on the plane and he hadn't thought to bring an extra shirt.

Here are some tips if you are planning a flight with your own little beasties and no adult backup.

1. Your kids will either view this as an amazing adventure, or a horrendous torture. If you are relaxed and non-stressed, they will be, too. Kids feed off your anxiety.

2. Smile at people. Realize that everyone looking at you is dreading a meltdown even more than you are, and they will be excessively grateful when your kids don't. Just smiling at employees has gotten me moved to the front of the security line, gotten extra snacks on the plane, and once gotten us invited into the cockpit of a 747 and allowed to sit in the captain's seat. When my seatmates realize they are in the third seat next to a toddler and a baby on my lap, I like to tell them that they won the seating lottery. This generally disarms them.

3. Every airline I have ever flown checks car seats for free. Tape your name and phone number to the bottom before you leave the house because there is nowhere to tie those ID tags to.

4. An umbrella stroller is a must for little legs under the age of five. I use it to carry the car seats into the airport, and also as a luggage cart. An older kid can ride on the back of an umbrella stroller (with the little one in the proper seat) until about age six. If your child is too little for an umbrella stroller, stack your carry-ons on the stroller, have the toddler ride on the back, and wear the baby in a baby carrier or sling. I kept Tiny Pants in the sling on the plane itself as a means of restraining him when he wanted to run all over the plane and taste things like armrests or other passengers. Strollers also work as high chairs once you reach your destination. You know those moving walkways that say "no strollers"? I ignore the signs. I am capable of managing to push an umbrella stroller on a moving walkway and even chew gum at the same time. No one has ever stopped me. (Don't sue me if you fall on your face, though.) I also yell "On feet" to the children at escalators, and the little guy jumps out of the stroller and I carry it on the escalator. I never have time to find an elevator.

5. If you have a second child walking beside the stroller, give them a designated spot. I tell the big one that my left side is his "spot." When I glance down in a moment of panic, I look in one spot, I don't have to scan both sides.

6. Wear a backpack as your carry-on. Single-strap bags tend to swing around and peg the older child in the head, and although backpacks are heavy, your hands will be occupied with the stroller and the other child and can't manage a rolling bag as well. Pack an extra shirt for everyone including yourself in the backpack, as well as three more diapers than

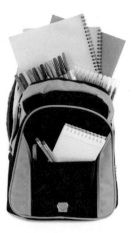

you think you need. Understand that your back-pack is not for you—give up on the idea of bring-ing a book or neck pillow. Go to the dollar store and fill your backpack with toys, activity kits, and food. Let the kids pack whatever toys they want in their own backpacks, but realize that on the plane nothing they brought will have any appeal to them at all. Their toy collection will have merit once you reach your destination, but on the plane, the toys are pretty useless. However, packing their back-packs the night before also keeps them entertained for ten minutes while you double-count the number of diapers in your own bag.

7. If you're lucky, your plane will have free in-flight movies, some of which are appropriate for children. There is something called a headphone splitter that allows you to plug two sets of headphones into one jack. They are amazing and cost under five dollars. If you don't have a split-ter, just give each kid one earpiece and remind them that movies weren't even invented when you were a child. Although some planes have out-lets under the seat, most don't, so your car DVD player will be useless.

8. Remember, it is you against them. This is the time to focus on survival, not nutrition. Be prepared to feed the kids every fifteen minutes, and I don't mean carrots. You don't want them to puke from too much candy, but bring things they won't whine about eating. On a two-hour plane ride, I have eight snacks. Also, bring an empty ziplock bag for all the sticky things you give them that they lick once and hand back to you. I once spent a very long twenty minutes holding two sticky lollipops and a wad of gum waiting for the plane to reach cruising altitude.

9. During takeoff and landing, the pressure change will hurt their ears if they aren't chewing/swallowing. If they are too little for gum, bring Skittles, Laffy Taffy, lollipops, or sippy cups. If they nurse, nurse 'em. People would rather see a boob than hear a baby scream every single time.

10. With children under the age of seven, avoid flights longer than two hours. You are better off with two shorter flights. Also, pay attention to flight times. You know your kids, and although mine are morning

people who love to leave the house at 5:00 a.m., not every child is like this. Bringing a child on a flight past their bedtime is asking for trouble.

11. Be prepared for the security line. Wear slip-on shoes and skip a belt. Kids don't have to remove their shoes anymore, but will have to remove coats. We leave our winter coats in the car when we are flying south. It's just not worth the hassle. When we are waiting in the security line I tell my kids that the security people are looking for hamsters in people's luggage. This reminds the TSA to be nice to the kids—they are small and easily scared. It always makes the screeners smile and be extra sweet to the kids. It also confuses the kids enough so they don't start thinking about real scary things they may be looking for; they spend the time trying to figure out why so many people bring hamsters on vacation. Also, talk to your kids about what to expect. They will have to walk through the metal detector by themselves, and they may freak less if they understand what is going to happen.

12. Note: I have never been asked to send the kids through the full body scan. They just use the old-fashioned walk-through metal detector.

13. Try to arrange for an hour layover between flights. Too much time will make you crazy, and too little will make you run too fast. If you miss your plane you will be sitting in an airport for hours. Detroit is the only airport I have even seen that has a play area.

14. When all else fails, play the squiggle game. It works for kids of many age levels and all you need is a pen and a bit of paper. You can do this on the edges of in-flight magazines or old boarding passes, in a pinch. It's very simple. You draw a squiggle, then the other person has to make a picture out of it. It's a great time killer.

15. Realize that when you land your children will be "done" but your relatives won't be. You have one job: get your kids fed and out of the car as soon as possible. They don't want to stand around jawing in the airport, or take the long way to drive by your old high school. They want their travel to be done, and now they need something healthy to eat or they will be sick to their stomachs and cranky.

16. One thing I occasionally forget is that the trip home requires the same amount of preparation. Now you have tired, worn-out children who have eaten all the snacks and used up all the surprises from the

outbound flight. Just because you bought them toys/souvenirs on your trip down does not mean they will be satisfied with this on the plane ride home. If you were smart, you brought return trip toys/snacks with you or snuck off to a dollar store while on vacation. If you are like me, you are now out of everything and considering hitting up the airport gift shop.

Note: Some of you don't believe in bribing children for good behavior. Some of you don't believe it is your job to entertain children or buy them surprises for trips. That is fine. You can also take some of the toys that are under the couch or otherwise long forgotten instead of buying new toys. You can bake cookies instead of bringing candy, and make them handmade travel journals to draw and write in, if you prefer. What you do need to do is have something novel for them, even if it is just a pretty shell or rock they can pretend is their pet. As long as you are mindful that travel is hard on little guys, that time moves backward on airplanes, and that nothing they own will entertain them and the flight attendant will bring you no food, you will be fine.

Recycled Snack Candy Bars

So now you have arrived back home after surviving two plane trips and a vacation with your toddlers, and you discover that since you were so focused on packing snacks and prizes and diapers, you neglected to plan for food when you arrived back home. While you assumed that you'd return to the house refreshed and full of energy and enthusiasm for household tasks, after waking up at 4:00 a.m. for your flight home you have neither energy nor enthusiasm and you are also out of snacks. What you do have plenty of are baggies of crushed pretzels/graham crackers/Goldfish that were at the bottom of your kids' book bag that no one will eat. If you also have wax paper and some sort of chocolate, you're in luck.

Ingredients
Wax paper
Bag of smashed snacks
Chocolate chips

Procedure
1. I bought wax paper for some art project I did with the kids—perhaps making crayon hearts out of broken crayon stubs or something that looked great on Pinterest and didn't work out so well in real life. I'm not entirely sure what went wrong—let's be honest, I'm never entirely sure what goes wrong between the concept and the execution of those Pinterest projects, but something

usually does. At any rate, I owned a roll of wax paper, which comes in handy every now and again.

2. Take a cookie sheet and lay a piece of wax paper on top. Don't crumple the edges down—it's just a resting place for it, not a permanent accessory for the cookie sheet to wear.

3. Dump out your baggie of pretzel fragments (or whatever snack in question) onto the wax paper.

4. Pour some chocolate chips into a bowl and put it in the microwave for one minute. OK, this is important. You have to stir every 15 seconds. For real. Chocolate chips have the weird ability to melt while still retaining their chip-like appearance. So while you look through the window, completely oblivious, the inside of the pile will start to burn, making a horrendous smell and wasting precious chocolate, which all divorced mothers know is a crime against humanity. So stir, even when they are still hard. Total cook time depends on your microwave. Mine took about 51 seconds.

5. Pour melted chips over broken snack item.

6. Pick up the long sides of the wax paper, and sort of roll all the broken things into the chocolate. Roll up like a burrito, but a very skinny burrito—about the diameter of a quarter. Thick chocolate/snack burritos are hard to cut. Let harden.

I know what you're thinking—*that's all well and good if your kid eats pretzels but my kid only eats crackers in the shape of fish!* Rest assured, fellow mama, this works just fine with smashed fish-shaped crackers, even the Xtreme Cheddar variety. At least, Tiny Pants thinks so.

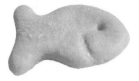

Tiny Pants and the Babies

The only real difference between having boys and having girls is the stuff you get to buy them—you know, all the stuff you wanted when you were a kid, but either your parents wouldn't spring for it or the thing just wasn't invented yet. I don't think I could love a daughter any more than I love my sons, so it's not that big of an issue, but having two boys meant I'd lost my opportunity to ever own a Barbie Dream House, or buy those sparkly tulle tutu skirts with the attached shorts, or collect baby dolls—or so I thought.

Tiny Pants wanted a baby when he was five years old—a real live one.

"Mama, I think you should have a baby and give it to me and Big Pants," he said.

"Well, what about when you went to Daddy's house? What would you do with the baby then?" I asked, somewhat sensibly.

"Oh, I'd bring it to Daddy's," he answered.

"I don't think Daddy would be on board with that." Daddy Pants wasn't a huge fan of the stuffed animals that went back and forth every week, so it was safe to assume a live infant wouldn't go over well, either. Daddy Pants had also been quite sure that two kids were all he intended to have.

"But it would be me and Big Pants's baby."

"Babies cry all the time. I think Big Pants would prefer a puppy."

"Totally!" Big Pants interjected. He had wanted a baby back when he was five, too, but he was over it.

"But they are on sale! We can just order one and go pick one up. See? I circled it in my catalog."

Sure enough, he had circled the baby posing with a toy in the advertisement several times. In sharpie. He meant it. I remembered back when I was trying to get pregnant how much I wished that Target really stocked live infants. It would have made life a lot easier. Still, even if one could buy a baby at the store, I wasn't planning on giving a baby to a kindergartener to raise. He barely fed the fish.

Big Pants had had a "Baby Brudder" doll back when I was pregnant with Tiny Pants. I hadn't purchased the doll for this reason specifically, but I still had my old dolls because I'm sentimental. Big Pants dragged Baby Brudder around for a few months, then eventually lost interest once his real brother arrived. Baby Brudder—for some reason renamed Baby Elephant after Tiny Pants was born—still knocked its hard plastic head around the bottom of their toy box, but its hair had turned into a plasticized frizzy matted hair-cap that was no longer attractive without a baby hat.

When shopping for Tiny Pants's sixth birthday, I came across a baby in the discount supermarket. For $8.88, we could own a doll with unrealistically (and slightly creepy) blue eyes. It said "nighty-night" and "I love you" in a cartoonish grown-up-woman-imitating-a-child-type voice. It giggled, and said not only "Mama," but "Dada" as well, plus it made Shrek-worthy burps and could be switched to Spanish if we so desired. If you were willing to clamp its head between your knees and exude a little force, the doll's thumb could be wedged in its puckered mouth. Although Daddy Pants was against Tiny Pants's doll lust, I figured the fact that it said "Dada" might make it more acceptable. (It didn't.)

On his sixth birthday, Tiny Pants stood on a dining room chair to better reach the pile of gifts on the table. When he ripped the paper off the box to reveal the orange and pink outfitted baby doll, his whole face lit up. I had made his birthday dream come true.

Tiny Pants loved his baby, but since he inherited my shopping tendencies, he soon wanted a better one—among other things, this doll was too skinny for real newborn clothing. My parents were more than happy to buy a new baby for Christmas. Lesbian grandmas are very good for buying princess costumes or any other gender-defiant toys that my children required. They spent hours searching online for the very best, most realistic baby that came equipped with the most gear—in this case, a bottle, a car seat, and a wearable baby carrier. Ironically, I'm not so sure they would have been so enthusiastic if I had a daughter who wanted a stereotypical toy of the patriarchy, but since I had sons, the grandmas were more than eager to provide a baby doll.

The new baby arrived in a blue footie pajamas with cow ears on the hood and a cow picture on the chest, so he spent some time being referred to as Cow Baby, then Cowie, but when Daddy Pants's aunt suggested "Carl" as a name Tiny Pants got mad and named it simply "Baby." (The original talking baby was loved but never named.) I realize that this doesn't sound like an actual name, but for some reason it was different from "the baby" or "your baby" as we referred to the first doll. Baby was much loved and went many places. He came to West Virginia for my graduation, to New York to see the grandmas, and Baby even went to Chicago to visit Daddy Pants's family.

Daddy Pants was not a fan of Baby, not even a little bit—in his mind, dolls were for girls and only girls. It didn't matter that Daddy Pants himself changed diapers, gave bottles, and raised the boys on his own a few days every week—that was somehow different. Daddy Pants's family seemed to agree, and Tiny Pants tearfully told me about his Chicago cousin (an adult) who threatened to give Baby a swirly in the toilet or lock him in the freezer. It broke my heart, but one thing about divorce that I hadn't really understood was how little influence you have when the kids are at your ex's house. There wasn't much I could do besides sending angry texts which went unanswered. Full disclosure: SigO doesn't love Baby, either, though he'd never put him in the freezer. He finds something unsettling about the unblinking eyes and permanent smile, and let's be honest, he worries about Tiny Pants getting picked on. I personally think that some kids are natural targets, like I was, while other kids, like Tiny Pants, have enough confidence and charm to be different and get away with it. Regardless, he might as well have toys he likes while he navigates the world.

My girlfriends and family loved and accepted Baby. My brother saved infant clothing that his kids outgrew. Mom friends who had girls gave me advice on how to remove the brown patina Baby was developing on his plastic face and arms, but Tiny Pants didn't want him cleaned. "He got some of that dirt on vacation," he explained. Tiny Pants was a hoarder by nature, but this sentimental attachment to dirt took it to an entirely new level. However, it turns out that plastic doll noses are incredibly hard to clean, so I was happy to have the excuse to give up on the process.

Baby was soft and huggable, but this made him not as realistic as a silicone baby, so soon Tiny Pants was longing for a new anatomically correct boy baby doll. He spent his free time watching videos of girls unboxing silicone dolls. They were cute, sure, but I wasn't about to spend over one hundred dollars on a doll when he had a perfectly cute baby already. I remained firm until Christmas got closer and I had no idea what to give him. I found a realistic (though neither silicone nor horribly expensive) baby boy doll that I thought was close enough. I went on eBay and searched for baby clothes. I lost my first two bids, so I got frustrated and bid on several lots at once. It turns out that bidding on multiple similar lots is a very effective strategy for winning all of them, so Tiny Pants got a whole suitcase full of baby clothes.

New Baby soon became known as Baby 2.0, and original Baby was renamed Baby 1.0. Baby 2.0 was much more realistic, but not as soft and huggable. Plus, his jointed arms were hard to bend when changing outfits, and we had to change outfits more times than I thought was necessary. We also had to change diapers nearly as often as if he were a real newborn—not because he pooped, mind you, but just because it had to be done. The next year, Tiny Pants wanted a Little Live Pets Snuggles My Dream Puppy for Christmas—no, the creators don't believe in punctuation, if you were wondering. I was willing to buy what I considered an overpriced, unattractive and potentially irritating toy in hopes that it would move Tiny Pants away from Baby 2.0. I'm a bad person, I know, but I was tired of defending Baby 2.0 to his father, and tired of trying to force his arms into tiny clothing.

Little Live Pets Snuggles My Dream Puppy was a disappointment. He was hard, due to his electronic body. He was loud and irritating to grown-ups. He didn't look much like a real dog. He was beloved for a few weeks, but quickly forgotten about. When we went to visit my brother and his family—which included a two-year-old adorable cousin—Baby 2.0 became beloved once more. Just as Tiny Pants started to lose his enthusiasm for his dolls, my sister-in-law graciously provided a second baby cousin, and we are now back into full-on baby-love, and secretly, I'm glad.

The truth is, I loved Baby, both versions 1.0 and 2.0. I no longer worry if kids will tease Tiny about his dolls. The part of me that loved and collected dolls when I was his age has reawakened. Tiny Pants and I email each other pictures of new dolls when he is at his father's house, and just last week we made a satin-lined bassinet together. Tiny Pants sewed the comforter and pillow all by himself. I know he will outgrow his babies soon enough—just like he lost interest in his Princess Elsa costume in favor of hockey pads—and I don't want to be that mother infantilizing her children. When it is time to put Baby 1.0 and 2.0 on a shelf I promise to accept it, but I may still have to give them a hug when the boys are with their father.

There's something else though. Tiny Pants went back to Chicago this week.

"Will you sew this baby hat before I go?" he asked me. It was a small, mint green baby hat my brother gave him when his ten-month-old baby had outgrown it, and it was a little too big for Baby 2.0. Tiny Pants folded the back of the hat to show me how much needed to be taken in. He dressed Baby 2.0 in a diaper, sleeper pajamas, and fleece body suit, and added the hat to keep him warm and well-accessorized.

"Am I watching Baby 2.0 while you are gone, or are you taking him with you?" I asked.

"Oh, I'm taking him," he answered, blowing the chin length bangs of his fauxhawk out of his face. He knew his cousins and aunts and father would likely tease him about Baby, but he put on his Harry Potter robe over his *Star Wars* T-shirt, picked up Baby 2.0, and that was the end of it. Somehow, I knew that he would be OK.

Oh Santa, I'm Sorry

I took Big Pants and Tiny Pants downtown to see Santa last weekend, as I do every year. We took the train as usual (which is quite possibly slower than driving, but more fun) but I messed with tradition just a little by using a different station. The new one was closer to our house, but it smelled like pee on the first floor and patchouli on the second floor. Big Pants voiced his opinion that in the decision of weird odors versus a shorter drive I chose poorly. I had to concede that his point was valid.

I watched the children closely, because I had a feeling that this might be the last year my kids would both still "believe." Tiny Pants wanted to know if the Santa we saw was an elf from the North Pole (my excuse for how Santa is in every mall across the country on the same day) or just a grown-up in a costume. I asked him what he thought because I'm the queen of avoiding difficult questions. Big Pants was quick to interject a theory about oversized elves that seemed well thought out and plausible. Big Pants still finds Santa completely rational. As I type this, he is working on a science fair project involving the laminar flow of air and other principles of physics I really only halfway understand, yet he blindly accepts Santa.

I worried just a little that I had let it go on too long. At what point should I say something? Or, was it possible that he knew full well about Santa and was just trying not to disappoint me?

(continued)

Nope. When we finally made it to the magical red lap Big Pants was a little awed by Santa. He was a bit intimidated to say what he really wanted for Christmas, but I gave him a nudge and he told Santa the only item on his wish list—a DNA test.

I was not sure if Santa understood that Big Pants wanted an ancestral DNA kit to learn whether his relatives really came from Germany as they claimed, or if they were, as he suspected, Secret Lithuanians. Suddenly I realized that the lack of clarity in the term "DNA test" combined with both the absence of a male parental unit in our family group and a naked ring finger on my left hand might cause a misunderstanding. Santa looked at me as if perhaps I wasn't a very choosy mom.

Tiny Pants had made a Power Point presentation for Santa, which he had printed out and stapled into a book, seeing as Santa's workshop was not all that technically advanced. Luckily, when Tiny Pants was reading his list to Santa, he substituted "real-looking rabbit stuffed animal" for "taxidermied rabbit" and didn't show him the photograph. I'm not sure Santa could have handled DNA tests and dead animals in the same photo session.

. . . .

Posted by Lara L Saturday, December 5, 2015 at 9:18 PM
Labels: Holidays, I Think I'm Funny, Not My Finer Moments

HUFFPOST
THE BLOG

Sometimes You Are Not a Victim—
You Are an Asshole

I have, for a lot of my life, suffered from a victim complex—you know the one, where everything in your life is someone else's fault. It is only now, a good six years after my second divorce, that I am starting to see how I was no treat to live with. Oh, I knew I had made mistakes, I just thought the other person had made more. We were both wrong, but I was clearly less wrong. Or was I?

Six Ways I Destroyed My Marriage:

1. A few weeks ago a friend came over. "What do you want for dinner?" I asked. "I don't care, whatever you want," she replied. I offered her several choices, all I was equally fine with. She still demurred.

   This was exactly how I was about every decision with my first husband. I thought the greatest gift was to have no opinions and go along with what he wanted. It turns out, when you are the one who always has to make a decision about everything, it's a bit of a drag. My ambition to become an amorphous glob of green Jell-O with no backbone, opinions, or suggestions made me one heck of a boring wife.

2. I was sick the other day. My significant other asked me if I needed anything, and of course I said no. Five minutes later I got up to get a glass of water, which I knew I wanted when

(continued)

he asked. Suddenly I wondered how many times I blamed people for not taking care of me when really I was obstinately refusing to be taken care of? I started to suspect that I wasn't just a victim, I was an asshole.

3. I was talking to a friend about her boyfriend recently, and she said, "He's so awesome, we never fight." This sent up red flags for me. I avoided conflict like the plague in both my marriages and it did not serve me well. Every time I said, "that's fine," when I meant, "that is completely not fine and we'll see how that works out for you," I created a chasm in our relationship, and my partner did not even have a chance to do anything about it.

    I always swallowed my anger, and that just allowed unresolved resentment to churn and grow until it took over everything, and I never even gave him a chance to stand up for himself or try make it right. I secretly seethed. Not very different from how I acted as an eight-year-old, come to think of it.

4. I love and hate to be touched. This is tricky. I crave physical affection, and I was quick to condemn partners for not being affectionate enough. It took me a lot of years and a new relationship to understand that I send a lot of mixed signals. For example, I love to have my hair stroked, but only in the direction it grows, except on the top and then only against the grain, and not too long in any one place, and please don't rub my head near my ears in the way that makes a crunchy noise in my cochlea and you didn't do both sides equally and why are you no longer petting my head? Men never pay attention to my needs, I thought. In retrospect I might have been a little bratty. I'm not sure I would have persevered if I were them.

5. I underestimated my ex's ability to change. I had a theory, coined in my twenties, that people don't really change for other people. If asked, they will exhibit new behavior for up to but not exceeding twenty-one days in order to appease you, then they will revert. If you don't like someone's behavior, you'd be better off leaving than expecting them to change.

My first husband was a high school graduate when I married him. I did not think he had the ambition to ever finish college, although he was taking a few classes here and there. Imagine my surprise when I learned that after our divorce he not only got his bachelor's but his master's as well—and years before I did.

My second husband became an organic health food nut, ran the Tough Mudder hard-core obstacle race, and learned to play guitar after we broke up—all cool things I never imagined he would have any interest in.

Certainly, they may not have changed if we had stayed married, but I never properly believed in their potential.

6. I was completely unwilling to compromise. My idea of compromise was we'll do it my way, I'll do all the work, and you won't complain about how I do things. I hated conflict and would do anything to avoid it. Unfortunately, by not fighting I created a dichotomous household. We stopped being a team and became two co-inhabitants, and not very cohesive ones at that. Relationships are built on compromise. It's part of the equation of sharing your life with another person, and forming that compromise teaches you something about yourself and the other person that is valuable.

Of course, there were many things wrong with both marriages, and I'm sure either of my exes would be happy to chime in on the myriad other ways I screwed up. Also, I'm not saying that I would go back and make a different decision, either, only that I realize that living with me was no picnic. If we cannot see our faults, we will perpetually repeat them, and I for one would rather make new and different mistakes this time around.

. . . .

Posted by Lara Lillibridge December 31, 2014 at 1:16 PM
Updated: December 6, 2017
More: Divorce, Learning from Mistakes, Relationships, Personal Growth

The Great Chicken Casserole Standoff

My biggest failure as a mother (so far) was what I like to call "The Great Chicken Casserole Standoff," or, as Big Pants calls it, "Casserole-gate." I was trying to find something everyone in the family would eat without complaint and break the boys of their dinosaur-shaped chicken and Easy Mac addiction. When it was just the boys and me, making them one thing and eating something else myself didn't seem like that big of a deal. I just opened the microwave, and everyone got what they wanted. Yet when we moved in with SigO, suddenly it seemed as if family dinners were important. Chicken casserole was one of the few things my mother cooked that I ate without complaint as a child, so it seemed like a good place to start.

SigO liked it. Big Pants liked it. Tiny Pants cut the world's tiniest bite, smelled it, and declared it unfit for human consumption. I asked him to eat a two-inch by one-inch serving. He declared that he didn't like 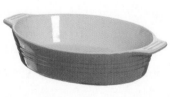 it, based on how it smelled and the most tentative of licks. I'm not even sure it counted as a lick—it was more like he pointed the tip of his tongue in the general direction of the casserole on his fork and it got scared and ran back to his mouth. At this point I made a colossally bad decision—I gave him an ultimatum. I haven't really done much with ultimatums as a parent, and I'm a bit of an amateur. Normally I relied on bribes, lectures, and threats so scary that they dare not be disobeyed, such as "I'll call Santa." But my parents used ultimatums and it seemed like the right thing to do at the time.

It started small. "Eat these two bites of casserole or else you'll get nothing else to eat tonight." When that didn't faze him, I escalated it to, "eat these two bites of casserole or you won't have any breakfast tomorrow, either." That got absolutely no reaction—no tears, no begging, nothing—so it became, "eat these two bites of casserole or you won't have anything else to eat until you do." Big Pants made a show of enjoying the casserole and asked for seconds, just to prove to his brother who the golden child was. (Big Pants is sometimes well-behaved because he is good by nature and sometimes well-behaved just to make his brother look bad.) Tiny Pants did not argue. He did not cry, beg, or cajole. He was completely impassive and started a hunger strike from dinnertime Saturday until he went to his father's at three o'clock Sunday afternoon. I begged, cried, and tried to entice him into eating those two bites. He silently refused and just went about his day, not even pouting or mentioning it again. Look—this is the kid I call "Snack Master Flash" because he eats every ten minutes. In no way, shape, or form did I expect him to successfully carry out a hunger strike lasting twenty hours. SigO thinks that we won, because we did not give in. I know that Tiny Pants won, because he didn't cave, either, and in the end, I was more upset about it than he was. Still, though, I hope he keeps that determination as he gets older. I think that unwavering steadfastness will serve him well in life—after he moves out on his own at least.

· · ·

If you want a very nice chicken casserole recipe that most people like, except for belligerent eight-year-olds, here is mine:

Chicken Casserole

Ingredients

Nonstick cooking spray

1 box Uncle Ben's Instant Rice (I'm partial to the wild rice, but whatever)

1 pound chicken, cut up into 1-inch pieces

½ bag frozen broccoli florets or cuts

1 can Campbell's Cream of Chicken Soup

½ bag shredded cheddar cheese

Procedure

1. Spray bottom of 9 x 12 pan.
2. Pour in rice, seasoning, and water according to the directions on the side of the box.
3. Add raw chicken (or cooked chicken, depending on what is in your fridge and how much time you have to kill) and frozen broccoli.
4. Stir in Campbell's Cream of Chicken Soup but do not add extra water. I know ignoring the directions on the label feels rebellious and wrong, but just do it. You can also use cream of celery or cream of mushroom if you prefer.
5. Add at least half a bag of shredded cheese. (Adults like things like pepper, but I don't use it because little black specks freak out the children.)
6. Cover with foil and bake at 350°F for 50 minutes to an hour, if you didn't use cooked chicken. 25 minutes if you did. If you are like me and never look at the clock when you put things in the oven, just wait a while and check to see if the chicken is still pink.

The Tooth Fairy Got Played

Last night Tiny Pants lost a tooth right before bed. I found the special tooth fairy box and we wrote the required note asking the tooth fairy to please, please let him keep his tooth, and put the note under his pillow and the tooth box beside the bed.

Thirty minutes later, good old Tiny Pants is bouncing on his bed and has "hid" his note for the tooth fairy on the floor in a little secret space between the nightstand and the wall. Clever, isn't he? I threatened to remove the tooth until the next night if he didn't go to sleep.

I set an alarm to remind myself, because last year the tooth fairy fell asleep, which caused all sorts of chaos and confusion. When the alarm went off, I snuck back into his room, dug the note out from under his pillow, and slipped the two dollar bills underneath. OK, shoved is perhaps a better description than slid, if you must know. Tiny Pants woke up but I got him back to sleep in under 3.3 seconds. Win.

This morning Big Pants woke up first. "I wonder if the tooth fairy left me anything?" he asked. *Scheisse!* When Big Pants started losing teeth, Tiny Pants was so jealous that the tooth fairy started bringing him a lollipop when his brother lost a tooth. It seemed easier. I had forgotten, or at least had hoped he had forgotten. He hadn't.

I ran back down stairs and rummaged through the cabinets for the new Dove chocolates I had bought (for myself) and ran upstairs

(continued)

with them cleverly concealed in my hoodie pocket. I very sneakily slid them under the folded clothes at the end of his bed I had put out for him to wear today.

Meanwhile, Tiny Pants was up and looking for his tooth fairy loot. The dollars were nowhere to be found. Look, I know I put it under his pillow. I was stone cold sober and in retention of all of my faculties last night. I did not dream it. But the money was gone. We took the pillows out of their cases. We used a flashlight to look in the crack between the bed and the headboard. We picked up the mattress completely off the bed. Nothing. Zip. Nada.

I ran frantically back downstairs, luckily found two more dollars in my wallet, and ran back upstairs. I fluffed his sheet and let the bills fall like little autumn leaves onto his bed. (Of course, neither child was looking at the time, which was a shame because my sleight of hand was Vegas-worthy.) Problem solved, or so I thought.

Tiny Pants commences to get dressed, and inside his UNDERPANTS beneath his pajamas he pulled out my neatly folded original two dollar bills. He was astonished. Or acted it.

"Four dollars Mama! I got four dollars this time!"

I think I've just been played by a six-year-old. I'm starting to look forward to the day they stop believing.

. . . .

Posted by Lara L Thursday, January 22, 2015 at 9:14 AM
Labels: Not My Finer Moments, Parenting, ToothFairyFails

The More Things Change, the More I Lock the Family out of the House

When I was married, I had three keys: house key, minivan key, and key to my then-husband's car. As soon as I left, though, my key chain quickly became cluttered. House key, minivan key, keys to the door of my new office job, key to my mother's house in case of emergency, key to best friend Asterisk's house in case of emergency, key to Herman's house in case of emergency, odd keys that I couldn't remember what they were for but didn't want to throw away in case they were important, and lots of those plastic loyalty store card thingies. I also had a detachable key ring that resembled a horse's snaffle bit, so I could detach half the keys if I needed to stuff them in my pocket. One side held the minimal house and van key (and also library card plastic thingie, because I always needed that) and the other half held all other keys required for general life and emergency purposes.

One November morning Big Pants had a field trip to Somewhere Exciting. The school bus left at 8:45, which was extremely important apparently, because the school had sent no fewer than three emails reminding me of the departure time, as if I were the kind of person that tended to be late, which I wasn't. I chanted, *"the Mama Bus always leaves on time,"* ad nauseam every morning. I felt scornful of the mothers who needed such ~~threats~~ reminders on field trip day.

I shook my purse to ensure that I could hear my keys rattling at the bottom of my bag and marched us out the door on time. As the door locked behind me I had that feeling that something was horribly wrong. I dug through my overly large purse that was filled with gum wrappers, Matchbox cars, a plastic watch Tiny Pants had filched from Asterisk's son that I had been meaning to return, a few small packets of lube I had been given at the gay pride parade over the summer that I kept because they made me feel adventurous, my wallet (of course), sunglasses, cell phone, and eight tubes of ChapStick. At the very bottom I found my keys. More precisely, I found half of my keys, because I had detached them the day before and thrown the half with my work keys in my purse so I wouldn't forget them in the morning. The front door to my house had a large window, and through it I could see the rest of my keys—the important half, with the house key and minivan key—looking dejected and abandoned on the stairway ledge.

I sent the boys into the back yard to play for a minute while I rattled the side door (locked) and tried to push up the kitchen window (foiled by the storm window) and called people to help. Nanny, my beloved babysitter, had a key to my house, but it would take her an hour to arrive, which would mean Big Pants would miss the field trip bus. I wasn't nearly as concerned about his educational enrichment opportunity as I was about being stuck with a kid all day when I had to be at work in an hour. Asterisk also had a key, but she had already left for her job downtown. "Mama, it's cold," Big Pants told me, showing me his little red-tipped fingers because his gloves were on the floor of the minivan which was also locked in the garage. I called the school about eight thousand times to beg them to hold the bus, but it kept going to voice mail. Next I called a married mom friend who was one of those super-busy "work two jobs and cook an eight-course dinner at night" type of people because she was effective, and I needed some effecting very badly right then. Super Mom laughed at me, but devised a plan. The children and I would walk a block to John's Diner, where we could wait in the warmth and eat toast. Super Mom would swing by (she lived thirty minutes away, and her daughter took the bus) and pick up Big Pants, delivering him to the bus. Tiny Pants and I would continue to play with toast (he didn't actually eat toast, but he liked to rip it into pieces) until Nanny arrived with the key, allowing me to liberate the minivan key and make it to work in something similar to on time. Although I was rather flighty about keys I was outstanding at my job and seriously underpaid, which hopefully would allow me some mercy from my very timely boss.

Super Mom managed to get through to the school's administrative assistant (I swear that woman really did have magic powers) and, still laughing, collected Big Pants as promised. She called me twenty minutes later to report that although he was the last one on the bus, he made it just in the nick of time. All his friends cheered and Big Pants gave high fives as he walked down the aisle of the school bus.

I would like to say that I learned my lesson, but I can think of two other times in the next few years in which I locked myself out of the house with the wrong side of my keys . . . OK, more than two times, but once Asterisk moved to my neighborhood, it became less of a big deal. Then it wasn't so much that I locked my keys in the house as that I just stored my house key in her silverware drawer.

● ● ●

When I moved in with SigO, my life became a lot less chaotic, and we hid a house key strategically in a box of car wash soap. I had bought it with good intentions but never actually used it to clean the car, because the children no longer thought washing the car was the best thing ever. I felt guilty about the waste of money, so it became my "mailbox" of sorts, where I stored a spare key.

That summer evening, the whole family went to the beach down the street to enjoy a picnic with some neighbors. We ran out of beverages, so the neighbor friend and I walked back up the hill to the house. Except the keys were still in SigO's pocket.

"It's OK, I have a spare," I told new neighbor lady friend, hoping she'd take the hint and turn her back. She didn't. I sighed and opened the garage door. She followed me.

"Oh, I bet you don't want me to see where you hide your key!" She said, one foot from my elbow.

"Yeah, actually I don't," I answered. She laughed but didn't move away. What could I do? I took the key from the car wash box and opened the door. I didn't put it back in the same spot, though, because now she knew where it was. While it was handy to have a neighbor who knew where the extra key was, she was a new friend with a teenaged son and I wasn't quite ready to trust her completely. That night, I hung the key up in the kitchen while I thought of a new and good hiding spot.

A few months later, we all returned to the beach to watch the sunset again. We got back home after dark with boys who needed to go to bed.

"I can't figure out which of your keys opens the door," SigO said, fumbling at the kitchen lock. *Oh fuck.* When SigO came into our lives in a cohabitation basis he brought a need for more keys. He had a winter home and a cabin in addition to the house we all lived in, and he had very sweetly and lovingly given me keys to all of them, which I kept on a carabiner hook. Except we had been at the cabin the week before, so he was holding the cabin and car keys, and the house key was on the key rack hanging gleefully next to the spare house key that I had not yet found a suitable place to re-hide. Did I say fuck? Yes, most certainly fuck. Luckily, I was complete shit at remembering to lock the back door—which apparently he knew, because he had double-checked and locked it himself. But we had had painters there that day! And they were painting the front door and probably were irresponsible and left it unlocked, and because we never used the front door, SigO had neglected to double-check it. Except the painters were exceedingly responsible that day and had locked it.

"I know the balcony door is open," SigO said, "I was up there with the painters and I know that I didn't lock it when we left." However, the balcony was on the second floor, and it was dark, and, while we are not exceedingly short people, we are also not ten-feet-tall people. Through some artful stacking of patio furniture and sheer determination, SigO managed to climb the pergola and pull himself fifteen feet (with a broken shoulder from Tiny Pants tackling him during touch-football a few months prior) across the wisteria and from there he shimmied over the rail onto the balcony.

"See kids? SigO is a man who gets things done!" I cheered, using my screw-up as a way to reinforce that their quasi stepfather was worth keeping around and also to underscore that hard work and determination pay off in life.

"Shit," SigO said from the second floor, "the painters locked this door, too. There's no way I'm coming back down in the dark."

So now I had two boys in the back yard and a boyfriend on the second-floor balcony and still no way to get into the house. Sure, I could call a locksmith, which was probably the best option, but two tired boys and one stranded SigO made the wait seem excessive when I had a brick. Which the boys were very excited to find for me, because they love to be helpful.

"I'm going to break the basement door window," I told SigO. Our house has a variety of doors, more doors, in fact, than any other house I have lived in.

"Isn't the dead bolt locked?" He asked. The basement door had a multipaned high-security-risk window, so it was also equipped with both a regular lock on the knob and a double-keyed dead bolt I was supposed to lock with a key, except I was lazy and perhaps too trusting of other people's laziness. "I didn't lock the dead bolt!" I confessed gleefully, for once proud of my lazy/flighty nature. Luckily, he didn't yell at me for my negligence. I have to admit that I was more than a little surprised that he agreed to my window-breaking suggestion, but he was standing on a balcony alone in the dark, after all.

I picked up the large gray rock my children had agreed was the biggest thing they could find in the garden. It was actually far superior to the brick I had planned on using, and besides, they were helping instead of crying or fussing. I had seen this breaking-windows-with-rocks-thing done in the movies many times. I took my fabulous favorite multicolored hoodie off and wrapped it around both the rock and my hand, to protect myself from breaking glass. I hit the windowpane closest to the door knob with the rock as hard as I could. Nothing. I hit it again. Thud. The movies made it look so easy. The third time I was rewarded with a cascade of broken glass (yay for me using the hoodie to protect my hand!) and I unlocked the door, then ran through the house letting everyone else in the family in.

The next day the very nice glass repair woman came and replaced the window.

"By law, we have to replace this with unbreakable safety glass," she told me. "So other people can't break in the way you did." I may be wrong but I think she looked at me like I was a complete failure at adulting. It was OK, I had already hidden the emergency key in a new location for the next time I locked everyone out of the house. We could say I had learned from my mistakes, but I'm still me, and that is unlikely.

Elephant Skin, Grinning Corpse Face, and Fighting Gravity

Let me just come out and say that I'll be forty-three this weekend. I'm not soliciting gifts or cake, I just want you to understand that when I say that the skin between my eyes is starting to resemble an elephant's knee, I'm not exaggerating.

This isn't a self-pitying blog where I'm zooming in on some tiny flaw and blowing it out of proportion for pity compliments. I'm losing elasticity. It's OK—it's age-appropriate. Not only that, but in the last year I've lost seventeen pounds. I only set out to lose seven, but then some of my remaining fat cells saw all their friends leaving and they followed them in solidarity. Or it was because I've been exercising six days a week for the last eight months and low-carb dieting. It could go either way.

The point is that all those happy little fat cells filled in my face and plumped up my wrinkles. My ass is high and firm but my face is slightly deflated. And while I could use this as an excuse to find balance through cupcakes and eat more carbs and fluff out my forehead, I'm in the best shape of my life, and I like how that feels.

Don't worry, this is not really an exercise blog. You can relax.

You see, gravity's a drag. Sincerely. (I've banned the word *literally* in my house.) It pulls your sternum toward your belly button and your shoulders toward your hips. It does very unflattering things to the skin on your knees and elbows. Still, since I started exercising, my posture is improved, and my upper arms no longer wave bye-bye after I've stopped moving my hands. I'm holding gravity at bay.

But.

Between my eyes I have the beginnings of an eleven forming, and of all my wrinkles, I find this pair the most appalling. Elevens are frown lines. Not only are they the scarlet letter of an unhappy life, but they also end in a stretched-out elephant-knee looking place between my eyes. You know what elephant skin is good for? Collecting oil and forming pimples. So my elephant-knee-between-the-eye skin has presented me with three tiny pimples for my birthday. I don't care for this even a little bit.

Yesterday I was in the car for five hours. The sun was shining and I was listening to an audiobook and drinking my energy drink and feeling pretty happy. I had no internet to convince me that the world wasn't a great place. And without the ability to do a word search puzzle or look for Pokémon or any of the zillions of ways I normally entertain myself when I'm alone and off-line, I let my mind wander. I also was doing isometric holds with my stomach and biceps in an effort to tone or stay alert, because it seemed like a thing to do.

I started wondering, if I can exercise my body by squeezing and holding a muscle, what about my face? I mean, underneath my middle-aged wrinkly skin there are supposed to be muscles, right? So I made the biggest grin I could muster while raising my eyebrows as high as I could in a surprised-corpse fashion. I decided not to care what other drivers thought of me. Besides, if they saw me again, in say the grocery store, I wouldn't be doing the surprised-corpse-grin thing, and therefore they wouldn't recognize me anyway. People tend not to notice your other features when you are grinning like a happy skull and driving by at seventy miles an hour.

(continued)

So I made the extreme happy face and held it for the count of five, then released. I repeated this over and over until I got to my destination. I noticed that my forehead felt tighter. My lips turned up at the corners when my face was relaxed. And if you have ever read any of that whole "fake it till you make it" type of advice, it really is true that smiling—even for no reason other than trying to reduce elephant skin—does make you happy. It's like I tricked my brain. In fact, I was so happy that I forgot to look in the mirror to see if it made a noticeable change, because one thing I have learned is never to use a magnifying mirror when you feel good about yourself, because it will do everything in its power to destroy any self-esteem you have.

When I finally got to where I was going, I picked up my SigO and we went to a party at the neighbor's place. The hostess commented that I looked glowy and beautiful and happy, which is exactly how I want to look, whether or not it actually improved my elevens.

. . . .

Posted by Lara Lillilbridge September 5, 2016 at 8:46 AM
Updated: September 22, 2016

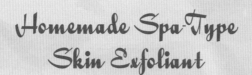

Homemade Spa-Type Skin Exfoliant

Ingredients

Small Tupperware container with lid (about the size that fits a can of Progresso soup. Not Campbell's, because you add water to Campbell's and that doubles the size of the Tupperware required. If you don't make soup, then a container about the size for a sandwich will do. Just an average one in other words, not a huge gallon-sized tub. Also, you won't be getting this back so don't use your favorite one).

½ cup baby oil (or olive oil)

Epsom salt

Procedure

1. Shake about an inch deep of Epsom salt into Tupperware container.
2. Pour oil on top. Mix.
3. While in shower, apply to body with fingers.

Mama (Accidentally) Makes a Dildo

Now that the boys are eight and eleven, I no longer make stuffed animals for them very often. Occasionally on a birthday I've been known to needle-felt a bunny or badger, but by and large it is an exercise in my nostalgia more than something they care about. At bedtime lately, though, Tiny Pants has been asking me for a "Mama stuffed animal," meaning a stuffed animal of Mama.

It's not actually his idea—a friend begged her child to go to sleep, and promised that if he did, she'd buy him any stuffed animal he wanted. The child replied that he wanted a "Mama stuffed animal" and then he would go to sleep. I thought it was a cute story and told it to the kids because I have no ability to consider the consequences of my actions, particularly when I'm tired. Ever since, Tiny Pants has been nagging me for a "Mama Stuffed Animal" of his very own.

I figured it wouldn't be that hard. I bought some iron-on transfer paper and took some selfies using my computer's webcam. Unfortunately, I didn't stand back far enough to include my feet. When you are creating what appears to be a voodoo doll of yourself with chopped-off feet it starts to feel a little ominous. I found a full-length picture of me, my brother, and our father that was taken recently, so I printed that out as well. Unfortunately, I'm the kind of person who looks incredibly awkward in forced poses, and I have this sort of wide-eyed zombie look that, combined with my giant smile, might just give my child nightmares. Since I was ironing it onto flannel instead of the flatter fabric the directions recommended, I figured maybe it would somehow magically blur just enough to work. Besides, my arms were at my sides, and thus I could make a really easy rectangular pillow thing that would still count as a stuffed animal, as opposed to the arms-and-legs-out-star-shaped selfie I had taken with the webcam.

I printed my selections, ironed them to an old flannel baby blanket, cut them out, and sewed them to some polar fleece backing for extra-snuggability, which happened to be pink.

Except when the background was cut away from the amputated-feet picture, the shadows had no relationship to any light source, and suddenly I had dark underarm areas that some might misconstrue as armpit bushes. Which they weren't. My mother didn't shave her armpits for my entire youth, so I became quite fastidious/neurotic about my own armpit hair. I've actually never grown it long enough to even discover its full potential.

I thought I had chosen wisely by wearing a long, flowy T-shirt so that I didn't have to hold my stomach in, but the flowiness made me look some-what larger than I am. The directions instructed me to leave about a quarter of an inch around the photo when cutting it out for a seam allowance. This added a teeny bit of extra width to my arms, and the background looked like part of my skin. It turns out, when you have just a little edge of off-white wall combined with weird basement lighting it gets a little vague. Did I really want to create lasting voodoo doll-esque art in which I appear chunkier than I am? Not, of course, that making your kid a doll of yourself wearing a skintight shirt would be good parenting. That's even creepier. It would have to be chubby mama or nothing. This wasn't about ego—it was love.

The zombie-eyed full-length Mama picture with non-chopped-off feet looked like my best option. Except that when I cut my brother out (sorry, Matt) I was left with a disembodied hand at my waist, which kind of com-plemented my undead gaze, but probably not in a way an eight-year-old would appreciate at bedtime. I sewed it together anyway.

The first thing I learned was that if you sew an iron-on transfer inside out and then flip it back right-side-out again (as is a common stuffed-animal-making process), it causes some stretching and wrinkling of the picture. This resulted in my skin looking rather elephant-like. I had hoped this might soften my zombie-stare, but sadly, it blurred my nose and mouth a bit, making my ~~slightly crazed~~ unusually wide eyes even more prominent. But that wasn't the worst of it.

Although the tube-like shape of the creation was as easy to sew as I'd hoped, I over-stuffed it in an effort to make the picture taut and unwrinkled. When one overstuffs a stuffed animal, the seams get a little bulgy, so now it looked like I had some sort of bizarrely disfigured arms. However, because my arms were at my sides and my head rounded the top, the final product most resembled a dildo. With my children's mother on it.

• • •

Even though my kids are incredibly accepting of my barely recognizable animals, I just couldn't bring myself to gift Tiny Pants with a zombie-mama-dildo-stuffed-animal. In the end, I wound up with the decapitated-feet mama doll that vaguely resembles a stingray. (OK, decapitated means cutting off of the head. *Pedibus* is Latin for foot, so technically I should say *pedibus*-itated but I somehow think the ~~sane~~ average reader wouldn't understand the reference. Besides, "decapitated" is fun to say.) And even though Big Pants has made no requests for a stuffed mama of his own, he'll be a teenager soon, and I'm sure he'll be needing a voodoo doll parent on at least one occasion. Or maybe I'll put a nanny cam in it with a microphone so I can eerily cackle, "Mama is watching!" when he tries to sneak a girl upstairs. So I made two lumpy un-footed armpit-haired slightly-chubby stingray shaped mama dolls for the boys and gave the dildo-looking thing to SigO so he wouldn't feel left out.

A Divorced Mom Talks to Her Children About Marriage

I had an unexpected conversation about marriage with my two boys yesterday. My eight-year-old thought that marriage vows expired every ten years and needed to be renewed. I think he got the idea from the 1990s TV show *Dinosaurs*, which we watch on Amazon Instant Video. I had to admit that I thought it might be preferable to the way marriage works now, and said as much.

"But then you'd be forced to live with someone for ten years before you could leave," my eleven-year-old objected when I voiced my opinion.

"Well, even now, in some cultures you have to live your entire life with the person you are married to whether you want to or not, until you die or they do," I retaliated.

"Why do you even need to go to court to get divorced? Just to keep lawyers in business?" my youngest asked.

"You need a license to get married, too. It's a legal contract, so if you want to end it, you have to go to court."

"If people got married forever, it might mean more," my eleven-year-old stated.

———————————

And thus my discomfort was complete. My kids know that I have been divorced twice. I'm sure that even having two visits from

(continued)

Santa is not always enough to make up for the fact that their father and I don't live together. Yet I don't want them to grow up thinking they are failures if they get divorced. I don't want them to think that they even have to get married. And I also don't want them to think happily ever after is just a pipe dream they can never achieve. This is the kind of important conversation I want to excel at.

Unfortunately, it is also the kind of conversation I have historically made a mess of.

"I'm not against marriage," I told them, which is true. "It's just harder than most people think it is before they get married."

That sounded lame, even to me.

"It's hard to know who you will be in ten years, or twenty years," I continued.

I knew that this thread was stupid, as my youngest hadn't even been alive for ten years yet. Fortunately or unfortunately, we arrived at their father's house, and the conversation ended.

This is what I wished I said:

Marriage can be a wonderful and beautiful thing. It can also turn your life into a pit of despair. (OK, maybe that's not the best way to broach the subject after all. Maybe I need to think about this a little more before I talk to my children.)

The truth is, I think our society does marriage backward. I think you should live your life with your beloved, raise children, fight, reconcile, cry and laugh and hug. I think we should go back to the idea of handfasting, when the wedding wasn't completely binding until a year and a day had passed. I think we should reserve elaborate wedding ceremonies for ten- or twenty-year anniversaries, when the couple has actually survived intact and they don't have to go into hock to pay for the party. We should celebrate the achievement, not the hope.

I do believe in commitment. I just don't think that it trumps everything else. I never want my children to think that they have to choose between feeling like a failure or being stuck in a life of wretched unhappiness. I want them to know there are other options—that they don't have to be ashamed to undo a life they thought they wanted but couldn't fit themselves into, but also that it is entirely possible to live forever with one person. And I want them to know that there is nothing wrong with never marrying anyone at all.

What I want is for my children to define their own lives, not constrain themselves to what they think is expected of them. I want them to find love—absolutely—but also know that they are enough on their own. They can marry a woman or a man or never marry anyone and still be successful in life. I don't care if I dance with them on their wedding day as long as I get to dance with them somewhere.

I sort of think that our relationships don't need to be celebrated by other people. I think buying friends and family members anniversary cards is kind of weird. I want my loved ones to be happy, but I have no say in whom they love or how they express it. I think it's a little odd to make a lifelong declaration of love in front of a roomful of people—it seems too intimate to share with others, like a first kiss.

So says the woman who had two big weddings with bridesmaids and the whole kit and caboodle. I recognize that it is easier to disdain that which I already had and rejected. I recognize that other people are entitled to the fairy-tale wedding if that is what they want. I concede that public declarations of love have their place in society, and I don't ever mean to mock those who find meaning in traditional weddings. It is only in retrospect that I feel the way I do now, though I was always flabbergasted by anniversary cards. College degrees and job promotions were

(continued)

achievements to be celebrated. Relationships are between the individuals involved.

Do I want my kids to get married someday? Honestly, I don't care one way or the other. Or to be more honest, my only hope is that they don't marry the wrong person, and if they do, I want them to know it's not the end of the world.

But I don't want them to lose that hope of happily ever after, no matter how bad at it I have historically been. They have every right to that dream, if they want it, and I will try my best not to be too cynical in front of them.

. . . .

Posted by Lara Lillibridge December 27, 2016 at 10:36 AM

Optional Items— Chocolate Cookies

One thing I have learned is that even if you don't have all the necessary ingredients, you can still make some sort of cookie. The other day the boys had a friend spend the night, so I decided to make cookies, because I generally make cookies any time the kids have someone over. Back when I was a little girl I resolved to be a Norman Rockwell–type mother someday, and while I fail at the housekeeping side of things, I do like to bake.

When I was still married I made homemade muffins for Big Pants every other day, using small $1 packets of premade mix that only made five muffins. Back then, I had things like required ingredients on hand, and if I didn't, I went to the store. After the divorce, I learned that a lot of required ingredients are more like suggestions. Also, children have low expectations when it comes to cookies. Tell them it is a cookie, and they will believe you.

I found a recipe online for cookies that used cocoa powder, because I had cocoa powder. I actually have no idea why I have cocoa powder, but for some reason (probably PMS-inspired grocery shopping) I had bought Ghirardelli cocoa powder sometime in the past six months. I did not, however, have chocolate chips.

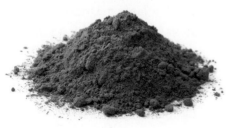

"Can you just smash up a Dove Bar?" Big Pants asked me. We generally do have Dove miniatures on hand, because they are an essential part of my not-killing-people life strategy, but unfortunately I had felt very stabby recently and had eaten all but one. One one-inch square of chocolate was not substantial enough to sacrifice for the cookies, and besides, I might need an emergency chocolate sometime in the immediate future, and it was best not to leave the candy bowl completely empty. I decided chocolate chips/chunks were optional. The recipe encouraged adding a cup or more of peanut butter chips, and I actually had some of those, but certainly not a cupful. Not even half a cup full, to be honest. I tend to eat them by the handful when the children are in bed. I figured I could just poke some in the top of some of the cookies, since Tiny Pants hates peanut butter anyway. I'd pretend that I only chipped half the cookies on purpose.

I was low on butter, so instead of using 1¼ cups of butter, I used ¼ cup butter and 1 cup of Crisco, because I had read somewhere that Crisco sometimes makes a better cookie, though I didn't remember why. Something about the spread or the chew or the airiness. I'd pretend it was on purpose. I mixed the sugar and assorted solid-state-fat together, but as I went to blend the cocoa powder, baking soda, and flour together, I learned that I did not have two cups of flour. I wasn't entirely sure what to do at this point, since the other ingredients were already mixed and it was too late to halve the recipe. Since I'm not yet at the stage of leaving the kids home alone, I decided to just see what happened.

"I'm making something resembling cookies," I warned the kids, "But I don't have enough flour, so I don't know how they will turn out. Just expand your definition of what constitutes a cookie."

"Will it be like a brownie?" Big Pants asked me.

"I have no idea what they will be like. It's an experiment."

I mixed in what little flour I had—it appeared to be around a cup—and hoped for the best. I spooned the "cookies" onto baking sheets and threw them in the oven, and the boys and I commenced to lick the various spoons and bowls. The batter was awesome. I looked in the oven, and instead of resembling cookies, the concoction had risen in a large gelatinous puffy manner, sort of like how I imagine soufflé looks in the oven. I have never actually cooked a soufflé, though, so that is merely conjecture. I consulted the recipe and learned this was normal. The cookies were supposed to do that, or something similar. The recipe assured me they would cool into something that looked more like cookies. Unfortunately, that meant we had to wait for the cookies to cool before eating them. I bake cookies for one primary reason—I love hot cookies and have no interest in eating them after they have cooled.

I watched the cookies cool while playing a video game on my phone. They started to resemble something cookie-adjacent, though they had morphed from circles into a large mass that had to be cut apart. I ate one, even though it hadn't cooled completely, because sometimes you have to sacrifice for your children. It was good. Very greasy, a little sugar-grainy, but definitely worth eating. I brought the cookies downstairs for the children, who devoured them. The next day, the mother of the child who spent the night told me her son raved about the cookies. It was as if I planned them to come out like that all along.

Here is my hacked version of the recipe I originally found on Food.com, though they might not want to be associated with it any longer.

Chocolate Cookies

Ingredients

2 eggs

¼ cup butter

1 cup Crisco

2 cups sugar (you can use 1 cup white and 1 cup brown if you run out of white sugar like I did, or any combination of sugar, according to my brother)

2 teaspoons vanilla

1-ish cup flour

1 teaspoon baking soda

¼ teaspoon salt

¾ cup unsweetened baking cocoa

Some peanut butter chips, if you have them. You could also use peanuts, walnuts, or chocolate chips, I imagine.

Procedure

1. Preheat oven to 350°F.
2. Mix together the eggs, butter, Crisco, sugar, and vanilla.
3. In another bowl, mix together the dry ingredients.
4. Now mix the dry stuff into the wet stuff.
5. Spoon onto ungreased cookie sheets, or just pour onto the cookie sheet, as they will all merge into one cookie anyway. Be prepared for them to double in size as they bake—don't overfill the pan.
6. Poke any chips/nuts you have into the top of the cookies, or don't. Up to you.
7. Bake 8–9 minutes.
8. Wait. They will turn cookie-like, I promise.
9. Feed to children, but probably don't try and sell at a bake sale.

ONLY MAMA

HOME | POSTS | ABOUT THIS BLOG | ABOUT ME

Clean Vehicle—Is That Even Possible?

SigO and I took an Uber the other day, or maybe a Lyft. I want to be accurate, but he was the one who called the car, and I'm not sure which app he used. It turns out that for the purposes of this story, it's irrelevant. I know what you are thinking—there goes six seconds of your life you'll never get back.

The point is that the Uber/Lyft car was immaculate. I don't mean just that it had been recently vacuumed. It looks as if no one had ever sat in it before. We chatted with the driver, as we often do, because it is really weird to sit in someone else's car and act like they don't exist. He admitted to having children similar in age to ours.

"NO!" I screamed. "Don't tell SigO that you have children!"

You see, I have been trying to convince him that the state of my vehicle is perfectly acceptable for people who have children. Sure, the windows are smudged with fingerprints, the floor mats are covered in baseball field dust, and there are a few gum wrappers and used tissues scattered around the back seat on any given day, but that is to be expected. My old vehicle routinely had random toys, empty food wrappers, the occasional dirty sock, and at least eighteen water bottles scattered in the foot wells. The children and I had *improved*. We had exhibited *growth*. This was the best that we could possibly do—except for vacuuming, which I intended to do one of these days, I promise—and also **the**

(continued)

best that all parents are capable of doing. The Uber/Lyft driver proved that cleanliness was obtainable, and there was no way, shape, or form that I wanted SigO to get that into his head.

"Do you make the kids ride on the roof?" I asked.

"I make them take their shoes off when they ride in the car," he explained. "They put their shoes in a bag."

This was *not* going well.

"And I have them trained to take everything out of the car that they bring into it as soon as they exit the vehicle."

Clearly, he was an alien, and had alien spawn children. Luckily, we got home before he could explain any more of his horrifying parental philosophy. Unluckily, we rode with a single mom friend the next week in her minivan, which was also impeccably clean. She was single—ergo, she was outnumbered by her children— and still her van was spotless. Her kids were five and nine years old—even younger than ours! I was betrayed once again. She actually apologized for not having recently vacuumed her vehicle, as if people actually vacuum vehicles more than once every other year! It was obvious that we can no longer accept rides from this woman, even if we are going to the same place. The cleanliness expectation level might get out of control.

Look, I know my car could be cleaner. To be honest, so could the house. Come to think of it, the children could probably stand more frequent washings as well. These are all things that I care slightly less about than I probably should. But I have many things in my brain that are much more interesting to me than cleaning and, sadly, often add to the disarray of the vehicle. Things like beach trips, Harry Potter festivals, drive-through safaris, and long relaxing car rides to visit relatives who live out of state.

The kids are very cute and I like them. I don't want to torture them more than necessary, and although conceivably there are parents who are capable of having happy, well-adjusted children and a clean vehicle at the same time, I am not one of them. We all know this.

The best plan I can fathom at this point is to carefully screen all potential Uber/Lyft/Friend vehicles ahead of time. If I get to the car first, I can throw some stuff around in there before SigO sees it.

. . . .

Posted by Lara L Saturday, February 18, 2017 at 9:30 AM

Labels: Not My Finer Moments, Parenting, Not Necessarily Single

Diamonds

I had a pretty good idea that I was getting an engagement ring for my last birthday. I had seen a jewelry store's phone number on our caller ID, and SigO said on more than one occasion that "I think I fucked up on your birthday present," and also "I think I made the biggest mistake of my life and I can't return it." Did I mention how romantic he is? Or how optimistic? I did what any good girl would do and surreptitiously started looking at wedding dresses online. Can I say that Google and Facebook ads—the ones that show you what you were last looking at but didn't buy—are extremely annoying when one is covertly looking at items like wedding dresses? I had a daydream or two about when and where we could get married. Not that I was in a rush or anything, but I grew up on Harlequin romance novels and Disney movies and my ten-year-old inner child was still romantically optimistic, in spite of my adult self's horrific track record when it came to marriage.

In spite of that, I was unprepared for what I felt when I opened that box. I did not know that one can simultaneously be captivated by a sparkly object and feel impending doom/panic at what it signifies at the same time. He was divorced (once). I was divorced (twice). I had already had three last names. And when he gave me the ring, he didn't clarify his intent by dropping to one knee or asking any questions. Finally, after slipping the ring on my finger by myself and pausing to admire the fact that he had purchased a ring correctly sized for my gargantuan hands, I had to ask him what conclusions I was supposed to draw from it.

"You know, in our culture, people have certain assumptions about diamond rings," I informed him, as if he were from Mars, or Antarctica, or somewhere else that didn't have diamond engagement rings. (Actually, they probably have engagement rings in Antarctica, come to think of it.)

"I wanted you to feel like you are as good as everyone else. I want people to look at you and know someone loves you," he said.

Sweet, but not shedding any light on this ring situation.

"So . . . are we engaged?" I asked.

"Do you want to be?" he asked. If he had clarified at this point that I could keep the ring regardless of my answer (as he had intended when he bought the thing), I might not have been so wigged out. The truth was that I did want to be engaged—sort of. I wanted to shop for wedding dresses, sparkly shoes, and white roses. But the idea that it would all result in marriage made me feel an urge to kick someone hard, and I figured kicking SigO right after he gave me a diamond ring might not go over well.

"I don't know. Do you?" I evaded. Scratch that previous comment—I no longer wanted to shop for wedding dresses. That was too real. I wanted to idly peruse wedding dresses online with the thought of "someday." Actually, the longer this conversation went, the less I cared about wedding dresses at all.

"Well, I'll marry you eventually, like before we die, but not right now," he said.

"I know you are my one true love," I rejoined. "And I really wanted a significant piece of jewelry, but the idea of getting married now makes me panicky."

"We both kind of sucked at marriage. But like if I got cancer or something I'd marry you. I mean, I'm sure at some point we'll do it," he said. This actually made me feel warm and fuzzy. He was talking like this whole wedding thing was something he did ultimately want—which was news to me—but thankfully, not now. The thought of a wedding this year (or even next) made me want to pace like a caged animal. If I had hackles, I would have raised them, yet another part of my mind was somewhere ensconced in tulle and satin ribbons.

"I won't marry you without a prenup," I clarified. "I want a guarantee that everything I brought into this relationship I can take back out again. That means the living-room couch, the guest bed, one car, and my savings account balance as of today. Plus, I don't ever want you to say I married you for your money. I want an ironclad document that proves I give no shits about your money."

"What about the kids?" he asked. "If we get divorced do I get any more right to the kids than I do now?"

"Nope." I was being honest—stepparents don't have legal rights after divorce, but also they are my kids and I already shared them with Daddy Pants and that was bad enough. I started thinking about what getting remarried and then divorced would do to the kids, and then I remembered that we had already been living together for over two years and the kids would experience a traumatic life event if we broke up now even if we never got married.

"But you know we're already fucked now," I clarified. "We can't break up anyway, because the kids are too attached to you. So we're kind of stuck together."

"We don't have to do it now. We can wait until we are really old," he added. "But I know that eventually we'll get married. And you wanted a ring, right?"

"I did want a ring," I agreed.

"So I guess you could call me your fiancé instead of your boyfriend," he said.

"Boyfriend is a stupid word when we are as old as we are," I agreed, "but fiancé sounds sort of pretentious. I mean, the word worked in my twenties, but in my forties? Come on."

"Betrothed?" he asked.

"I can live with betrothed," I said. "It sounds kind of cool."

• • •

Explaining it to the kids was easier than I thought. I figured they'd notice the diamond and ask—they didn't. They were used to Ring Pops, after all, and this was nowhere near the size of wearable candy. I thought they'd wonder what SigO got me for my birthday—they had no curiosity at all. On the way to drop them off at their father's, I figured it was time to gather my chutzpah and say something. Besides, it was always easier to talk when driving, as I didn't have to make eye contact.

"I want you two to hear all the important family news first," I began. "And people might say something when they see the ring SigO got me for my birthday, because diamond rings have a special meaning in the United States, and someone might ask you about it." I glanced in the rearview mirror. No noticeable interest.

"Can we play Pokémon Go?" Tiny Pants asked.

"Not yet. I'm trying to talk to you. This is important. I guess you could say SigO and I are officially engaged. But we aren't getting married this year. Or anytime soon. But eventually we will."

"Is it because you are sick of saying boyfriend?" Big Pants asked.

"Well, that's part of it, but I'm not sure fiancé is better," I said.

"That sounds dumb too," Big Pants agreed.

"But you could call him your future stepfather now instead of your quasi stepfather if you wanted. Or not. Whatever."

"Can I have a big sparkly ring, too?" Tiny Pants asked.

"You gotta find someone to marry you first," I started to say, but stopped myself. "Sure you can, once you get a job and save up your money. You can buy yourself the biggest ring you want." That sounded better, right?

• • •

The day after we officially got engaged, I was actually early to pick up the kids from school. I hovered in my car, next to a mom acquaintance also hovering in her minivan. We half-rolled down our windows and chitchatted while we waited.

"Wait, are you engaged?" she asked. How had she possibly noticed my ring through two car windows? Oh, right—she was a single mother, too. Single mothers always notice left hands, remember? "I thought you were all into the alternative lifestyle and were never going to get married again?" she asked, sort of hostilely. Or maybe she said it quizzically and I was just defensive, because I had indeed spent years not only saying exactly that but also writing blogs and essays declaring my refusal to buy into the marriage system again.

"Well, we aren't ready to set a date. We're engaged in that 'someday we'll get around to it' kind of way. And the 'I really like jewelry way.'" I said.

"I get that ring thing for sure. And hey—now you don't have to say boyfriend anymore! You can say fiancé!" she said, and then it was time to start our engines and roll up our windows and pick up our little urchins, I mean darlings, from school.

Italian Wedding Soup

SigO introduced me to Italian Wedding Soup at a small restaurant that served it in tiny white cups. I didn't want to try it—not even a little bit. I didn't think meatballs belonged in soup, and besides, it had both spinach and ugly noodles in it. While I understood that pasta tastes the same regardless of what shape it is, I found these particular noodles to be aesthetically displeasing. They looked like someone had taken ziti and chopped it up with scissors. But since I didn't want SigO to notice that Tiny Pants might have gotten his picky eating genes from me, I bravely tried his soup. I liked it so much I ordered my own, and now get it every time we go to that particular restaurant. I even eat it at home on occasion. Since the previous chapter involved engagement rings, it seemed like the proper recipe to include.

1. Buy Progresso "Italian-Style Wedding Soup." Do not ever buy low-sodium soup, and I wouldn't waste my time with off-brands. I've had that go horribly wrong before.
2. Heat soup in pan, pour into bowl.
3. Float one slice of Swiss cheese on top. Bring rest of the package of cheese to the table, so you can re-cheese the soup after the first slice is gone. After all, cheese is love.

HUFFPOST

Saying Farewell to the Tooth Fairy

The tooth fairy was the latest casualty in our household. Now, I have a love-hate relationship with the tooth fairy. There was the time the tooth fairy fell asleep, and the time the tooth fairy got played. I have long felt as if the tooth fairy was the least believable of the Childhood Magic Crew (CMC). I mean, why would she want a tooth in the first place? And why are teeth so valuable? Is she recycling them somehow, and giving them to other children in need? Planting them in the backyard and growing humanoid creatures to do her bidding? It's best not to think on her motives too deeply.

I was tired of the charade. The Pants brothers are getting a little old. I don't want them to actually believe in the CMC anymore—I feel as if they've outgrown the concept—but I don't mind them playing along with a wink. But that's not exactly how it went this week.

Big Pants, now an eleven-year-old, lost a tooth. For those unfamiliar with the tooth-losing patterns of childhood, they lose a bunch, then go for long spans without losing another. When Big Pants got a wiggly tooth, he found it annoying. I couldn't tell if he was also a little excited about it in that Christmas is Coming sort of way. (Not that the tooth fairy gives much in the way of cash in our house, but still.) Mostly he just wanted it out so he could move on with eating crunchy things.

Big Pants: My loose tooth is making me crazy!

(continued)

Me: Maybe you should just yank it out.

Big Pants: I'm playing dodgeball later. I'm sure I'll get hit in the face a couple of times.

Unfortunately, dodgeball didn't do the trick. Neither did baseball, basketball, or any of the -ball words. Biting into a slab of chocolate in the car worked nicely, but when he got out of the car, he instantly dropped the tooth in the driveway, and although we half-heartedly looked for a while, it was never found again. (There are apparently a lot of tooth-sized whitish pebbles in our driveway.)

That night he went to his father's, so the tooth fairy or no tooth fairy debate was out of my hands. Mostly. His father chose not to do any sort of tooth fairying. No judgment—the kid is on the cusp between big and little—but the problem wound up back in my lap.

———————————

Me: So Daddy didn't do any tooth fairy thing?

Big Pants: He just handed me cash.

Me: Do you still believe in the tooth fairy?

Big Pants: I don't know. I haven't lost a tooth in a couple of years. I haven't thought about it.

I retreated. Did I let him grow up, or did I encourage the charade? Did we need to continue the magic for his nine-year-old brother? I love magic. I am tired of playing tooth fairy.

I went outside and discussed it with SigO. We hemmed and hawed. Surely, he must know the tooth fairy isn't real. Certainly, he wants cash, which his father already provided. We looked for the tooth again slightly more than half-heartedly, but not full-heartedly because it was raining. Once again, we couldn't find it. I went back inside and dragged Big Pants's attention away from his Chromebook for another discussion.

Me: I looked for the tooth again, and couldn't find it. We could draw a picture of the tooth if you want.

Big Pants: It's okay, Dad gave me money.

I didn't pursue it further. This morning I woke up and wondered if I should have preserved the magic with a wink "for his little brother" who is not actually so little anymore, either.

But I didn't want to start a tooth fairy multiple-household tradition for the rest of the baby teeth in the household.

But I want to let him grow up.

But I rarely have small bills in my wallet.

But my house is slightly less magical than it was last week.

I guess I wasn't quite as ready to give up on it as he was.

. . . .

Posted by Lara Lillibridge June 15, 2017 at 9:28 AM

How I Became a Hockey Mom Against My Better Judgment

I walked into the hockey rink at 6:30 a.m. on a Saturday. Now, drop-off for school didn't even start until 8:00 a.m., so 6:30 was not a time I was normally awake, nor was it a time I wanted to be awake. The coach had promised to bring coffee, but I didn't see anything resembling coffee anywhere and the concession stand was closed, because the people who ran concessions were home in bed—where all good people belonged at 6:30 a.m. on a Saturday. I hadn't intended on becoming a hockey mother.

Unlike when I signed Big Pants up for travel baseball, I knew exactly what I was getting into when I signed Tiny Pants up for hockey. My first-ex-husband's nephew played hockey back before I had children, and I knew all about the crack-of-dawn practices, out-of-town tournaments, excessive fees, and let me say once again—practices at the bloody crack of dawn. So how had I wound up at a rink at 6:30 on a Saturday?

• • •

Tiny Pants was an extraordinarily happy baby—above and beyond normal baby happiness—but all that ended when he started kindergarten. He was excited to finally go school with his brother—they were two years but three grades apart, so he had been waiting what was felt like forever to a five-year-old. Tiny Pants wore a school T-shirt and navy blue dress shorts every day all summer long. He got a new haircut and one of those scuba-material lunch bags with pastel-colored owls all over it, and we added iron-ons with his initials. The school did a cute and ill-advised morning program with all the parents—we took pictures, heard a story, and walked out of the room to the sound of our children—including Tiny Pants— sobbing. They should have known better—it is easier for young children to leave their parents than to watch their parents leave them. This is why the Montessori school retrieved the children from the cars one by one, so the children walked in without looking back.

After Tiny Pants's heart was broken by watching his mother abandon him, he quickly learned that kindergarteners and third graders don't inter- sect in the halls at all. Big Pants was on the second floor; Tiny Pants's class was on the first. They didn't see each other except in the pick-up line after school, and maybe once or twice in the halls in passing. And someone made fun of his lunchbox.

Every morning we'd pull into the drop-off line at school, and every day Tiny Pants would start to cry and my heart broke into a thousand mama-shards. We made it through kindergarten and first grade. We went on playdates with kids from school. I volunteered in his classroom once a week—something I was not a huge fan of but felt was important. When I entered the room, a bunch of small people came running at me and hugged my knees, while my own beloved small person sat quietly in his seat. "We're not supposed to run around the classroom, Mama," he told me in explanation.

I offered to sign him up for any clubs he was interested in. He picked a creative writing class and wrote heartbreakingly sad poems. Now, one of those poems won honorable mention in a national contest, but I'd rather a happy child than any prize—even one for literary merit. I had to do some- thing to save this kid. I asked him of all the possible activities in the world that he could sign up for, what he thought would make him the happiest. He chose hockey. I was slightly less than enthusiastic.

• • •

"We have to save that kid. If he wants to play hockey, let him play hockey," SigO said. I called the local rink and learned that although it was November, I was several months too late to sign up for hockey. I called the rink in the adjoining suburb, and learned their practices were inconvenient—Daddy would have to take him Mondays, and I'd take him Saturdays. I started to tell the nice woman that it was unlikely that he could make regular practices on Mondays as his father lived a half hour from the rink and it was a school 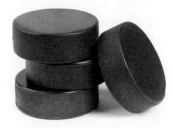 night. She interrupted my "thanks, anyway!" attempt to escape my fate with the words, "we will make it work. We want every child who wants to play hockey to be able to play."

Fuck. I had no remaining excuses. The kid already knew how to skate, thanks to two sessions of lessons and a neighbor who had installed an ice rink in his back yard. Daddy Pants even reluctantly agreed that it was in the best interest of the child. I reluctantly went to the store and bought a full set of slightly used hockey equipment.

Now, everything comes easy to Big Pants: school, baseball, science fair, math team, guitar, mock trial. Tiny Pants learned to crawl, use a fork, and tie his shoes at an earlier age than his brother, but that two-and-a-half age gap meant that Big Pants still did everything first. By the time Tiny Pants was big enough to participate Big Pants was more skilled—except at hockey. Tiny Pants can outskate him. The fact that Big Pants is unable to stop on ice skates without crashing into the boards makes Tiny Pants smile, though he tries to teach his brother how to do a hockey stop and raise a shower of ice. Sure, Big Pants could excel at hockey if he played regularly, but I won't let him play hockey, too. Tiny needs something that is all his own.

I've made new hockey-mom friends, learned to keep a warm blanket in the car at all times for cold ice rinks, and I have even rung a cowbell in the stands during a tournament. I've learned to air out equipment promptly and not to cringe when my kid gets checked by someone bigger.

He no longer needs me to help him get dressed, though I still strap his pads on his legs most of the time. *This will be the last year of this*, I think as I help him transform from my sweet, skinny son into some sort of armadillo creature. Pretty soon, it will be *no moms allowed* in the locker room. Pretty soon, he will be impatient with my helping. His greatest joy this season was breaking his stick during a game.

My biggest challenge so far, though, was running the time clock. I hadn't meant to volunteer, because I am inherently lazy, love kibitzing with my mom friends during games, and really suck at paying attention. I am the mom that never knows the score, and sometimes doesn't even notice the game is over until everyone else stands up. Time clock operator was a bad fit for me. However, I opened my mouth to say no, and "sure" came out. I blame that not-paying-attention thing I mentioned earlier.

Here's the thing about hockey families, in case you are unfamiliar. They are pretty intense and not afraid to get loud. Here's the thing about me—I am easily intimidated by loud, intense people, and also not very good at paying attention to things like goals and time clocks. What could go wrong?

I was provided with a diagram explaining the operation of the time clock. Now, normal people like diagrams, but for some reason diagrams fill me with unmitigated anxiety and confusion. I have been brought to tears trying to assemble a Big Wheel bike. When I was married, I just handed over all diagrams to whatever husband I was married to and let them figure it out. I didn't mind helping, mind you, I just am not good at decipher-ing pictographs. Words, people. I'm good-ish with the words. However, I came to the rink equipped with a secret weapon—Big Pants. He loves diagrams, contraptions, and paying attention at sporting events. Also, loud scary hockey people don't yell at preteen boys as often. I was saved!

After sitting in the box with Big Pants twice, I decided that I could do run the clock on my own when he had a cross-country meet. This was fool-ish. Remember that paying-attention thing I said I wasn't good at? It turns out that sitting next to someone running the time clock does not actually teach you how to run a time clock. I thought I had it down, and luckily, it wasn't a high-scoring game. A few times I lost track of whether I had hit the buttons already or not, but there were people to remind me. Then the period ended. When the period ends, the clock automatically runs out and a buzzer sounds—I didn't have to hit the buzzer button or anything. Easy. But right after the end of the first period is the second period, which requires that everything be reset again and which I had forgotten how to do in the twelve minutes since I did it the first time. I hit a button. *EEEEEE* the time clock responded. MUST CLEAR TIME OUT, its display read. Clear what? I hit ESC. *EEEEE*! I tried to hit "new period." *EEEEE!* Someone ran over with the Zamboni driver in tow. He admitted that he had no idea how to run the time clock, either. *EEEEEE!* I hit random buttons until the noise stopped and the clock reset itself, which was awesome and appreciated but I had gained no knowledge in the experience. Twelve minutes later, the second period ended, and once again, the refs, players, and fans had to wait while I kept hitting buttons and the clock kept yelling *EEEEE* at me. Finally, I realized what I had missed both times (and was not on the diagram): I had to toggle the ON ICE lever thingy which I had assumed magically reset itself when the buzzer went off.

I was never going to volunteer to run the dang thing again, but apparently no one else wanted to run it, either. After watching the sign-up sheet remain empty all week, I clicked "sign up," even though Big Pants would once again be at cross-country practice. It turns out the intense fear of the time clock has the same adrenaline rush as a roller-coaster ride, only without having to stand in a long line first.

ONLY MAMA

HOME | POSTS | ABOUT THIS BLOG | ABOUT ME

Freudian Lawn Job

I accidentally drove over Daddy Pants's lawn when I dropped the kids off yesterday. Not his whole lawn—just the edge of it right by the driveway. I'm sure he noticed—my ex was meticulous about lawn care when we were married to the extent that I was forbidden to mow the lawn. (Thank God.)

I didn't even notice that I was on the grass until I exited my vehicle, and he was already outside. I'm kind of not very aware of the edges of my vehicle, as evidenced by the scratches and dents I collect going in and out of my own garage, which, let's be honest—my ex probably notices as well. (Note to self: actually call body shop this week.)

What's even worse is that this was not the first time I have driven across my ex's front lawn. Nor was it the second time. I pretty much drive over his lawn every single week, which might account for his taciturn attitude. We are both conflict avoiders, and his silence blankets both of us, so I don't say I'm sorry, though I want to.

I want to explain that the reason I always nick the grass is that I am trying too hard to be accommodating. I am compulsively early, and at least a quarter of the time I arrive to the drop-off before he does. I want to make sure my ex has plenty of room to pull into his garage, so I stay to the left, only just a little bit too far over.

I am aware that this used to be my side of the garage and therefore driveway, but since I left, my ex parks in the middle of

(continued)

the two-car garage. Maybe that's why I feel the need to scrunch over as much as possible. He has rewritten his life without me, and when I intrude, I can't seem to help make a mess of things, or at least the lawn. Maybe it's just that since I left there's no room for me in any part of his life, not even the driveway. My SUV reminds me that I don't fit here—let's be honest—that I never fit here. I was always hopeless at staying inside the lines.

Every week I vow that I will be more careful, and yet the next week, I again pull too far to the left and end up in the grass. On good days, it is only the front tire. On bad days, it is both the front and rear. Maybe I unconsciously do it to provoke him to finally speak. Maybe I do it to make him glad I left. Maybe someday I will learn to keep my vehicle to myself, and stop driving over his lawn. (Oh, hell, even I know that is never going to happen.)

· ·

Posted by Lara L Monday, May 29, 2017 at 9:30 AM
Labels: Not My Finer Moments

For the Love of All That Is Holy, Can We Please Agree That All Women's Clothing Needs Pockets?

Do you know what I'm outstanding at? Going to the store and forgetting everything I went for in the first place. I lose lists and coupons between the kitchen counter and the store. Every freaking time. It's a gift, really. I mean, my ability to lose things is above and beyond the common person's—I have raised it to an art form, complete with pocket-smacking interpretive dance. However, the advent of the list app on my smartphone has made me more efficient, because I rarely lose my phone. Well, I rarely lose my phone as long as I have pockets. I always lose my phone if I don't have pockets, which is why I have worn the exact same Levi's denim skirt almost every day this summer. It has man-sized pockets. They are so roomy I can actually sit down with my phone in the front pocket and get my hand in there to retrieve it when it rings—or when I need to read a text. Let's be honest, the only thing I want to do when my cell phone rings is hit it with a hammer. I'm not a talking-on-the-phone person. We used to just call it a "phone person" but now phones do so many other things besides forcing you to talk to your relatives. I call mine "the pocket googler" because that's really its best use—not that I'm above playing word searches, reading with my Kindle app, or listening to audiobooks on it. I text people and am constantly on email and Facebook and Twitter. So I'm a phone person, but not a talking-on-the-phone person.

Back to pockets. It used to be that phone clips were cool. It didn't matter if you had pockets or not—you could just clip the phone onto nearly anything. Not dresses, and not things that were lightweight and stretchy, but everything else. Benefit of the phone clip:

1. You never sat on your phone,
2. Your ass didn't have a giant rectangular phone blocking it from view on first dates, and
3. You could buy clothing without pockets, which was good because women's fashion designers hate pockets with a vengeance.

Designers hate pockets more than I hate snakes or my children hate vegetables, and I hate snakes quite a lot. Okay, I don't really hate snakes, but I am afraid of them. I mean the screaming and running kind of abject terror that is completely irrational and not at all dependent on the snake being large, venomous, or able to make scary sudden movements. So I guess "as much as I hate snakes" is a bad analogy. However, my children certainly hate vegetables. Tiny Pants smells them to decide if he is even willing to lick them, and if they don't lick right, there is no way in hell that he is going to bite them. That's the way fashion designers approach the pocket. They sniff it, consider licking it, and most often back away in disgust without really ever fully contemplating the pocket. I have accidentally bought cardigans without pockets, skirts, pants, and shorts without pockets, but when I saw a winter jacket without pockets I decided to go on strike and refuse to buy another single item of clothing that was pocket-less. Thus, as I said, I wear the finely pocketed Levi's skirt nearly every day, except, apparently, this one. Since I had no pockets, I lost my phone and went to the store without it. Without my phone I had no idea what I was supposed to buy, and thus forgot taco seasoning on taco night.

By the way, if you lose your phone in your house, you can google "find my phone" from a laptop, and it will ring your phone at an incredibly irritating decibel level and won't stop until you answer it. Unfortunately, you cannot google "find my taco seasoning which I thought I bought but

I guess I didn't and now am in dire need of because the meat is on the stove already and I can't back out now." Turns out there is no app for that. There are, however, many recipes for taco seasoning online. Because I'm adventurous, I mixed and matched several recipes based on what I actually had in the cabinet that seemed to make sense. It worked, if you like burn-your-lips-off hot food, which I do. I didn't until after Tiny Pants was born, incidentally. I think perhaps my labor screams deadened the nerve endings in my mouth.

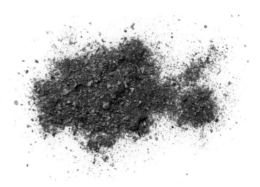

Fiery Taco Seasoning Mix

Ingredients

1 tablespoon chipotle chile powder (normal people probably use regular chili powder)

¼ teaspoon lime, garlic, and cilantro seasoning (They sell this all mixed up in one bottle. I didn't have plain garlic powder, and I figured cilantro and lime sounded like things that belonged in taco seasoning. I mean, I think they are in salsa.)

¼ teaspoon minced onion (for those of us who don't have actual onion powder)

¼ teaspoon crushed red pepper flakes

¼ teaspoon dried oregano

½ teaspoon paprika

1½ teaspoons cumin, which I thought was from India, not Mexico, so I had to google it. Turns out it is from the Middle East originally, but then again, traditional Mexican tacos don't use red and yellow packets labeled "Taco Seasoning" either, so who cares?

1 teaspoon salt. Really. I tried with half a teaspoon because who the hell wants to eat a teaspoon of salt? Apparently it adds some sort of taco magic because it didn't taste right until I added the rest of the salt.

1 teaspoon black pepper

Procedure

Mix together in bowl, add ⅔ cup warm water, mix again, then pour over your ground beef while it is still in the pan. I assume you know the rest of the taco procedure already. If not, consult the box of hard shells; it has directions thoroughly written out. The recipe was for taco mix, after all, not entire tacos.

The Family Blender

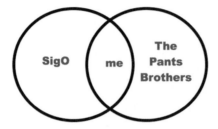

I often feel as if we are more of a Venn diagram than a blended family.

Due to shared parenting, nearly half the week SigO and I function as a childless couple. We have friends who have never met the children. The rest of the time, my focus is on the children. Sure, SigO helps with homework and we all eat dinner together every night, but I take them to all their lessons/games/museums/amusement parks myself, both because the kids like Only Mama time, and if I torture SigO too much I might run him off. Every now and then he comes along, but in general he doesn't enjoy kid things and I don't want the kids to feel as if they are constantly sharing me.

I've been slow to share authority with him. My mother gave complete control of discipline over to her partner, and we hated her partner for it. We never had a chance to develop the warm relationship with her that my mother hoped for, mainly because she was always the bad guy. My refusing to allow SigO to be a complete co-parenting partner is a knee-jerk reaction to my own childhood. And we fight about it on occasion. Don't get me wrong—he and I always come to an agreement on rules we can both live with, but I'm not exactly a peach about discussing it. I often feel as if the boys and I are an orbit of three planets, and SigO is a satellite in my gravity field, but not the children's. Yet everything goes to hell when SigO goes out of town.

• • •

"If you need me, I'll be in my room, right at the bottom of the stairs, with the door open," I told the children. "I'm just going to let the dog out and grab my computer." We'd already run thirty minutes over Official Bedtime, and still the children didn't seem anywhere close to ready for bed. I went downstairs, and our black-and-white dog was rolling all over the terracotta-colored family room rug. I think vacuuming more than once a ~~month~~ week is excessive seeing as the dog only weighs twelve pounds, and yet my just vacuumed carpeting was covered with a snowfall of dog hair. I hooked the dog to his tie-out and went into the kitchen to refill his water bowl. On the edge of the hardwood floor, slightly overlapping the carpet, was a warm pile of mush that had recently been inside the cat.

When SigO's gone, the kids wake up frequently and don't seem to have any faith in my ability to protect them from nighttime monsters. Honestly, I don't entirely blame them. It's been four years since I've been the sole defender of the household. I surround myself in a nest of pillows and sleep with a night-light on when SigO is out of town, so how can I get upset with the children when they can't sleep, either? But what it tells me is that in spite of any perceived distance, they rely on SigO and feel more secure when they know he's home, even if they are off playing elsewhere in the house. Everything is smoother when he's here—the children go to bed on time and the dog remains in his basket, where he snoozes and farts happily. The cat—OK, I can't lie, the cat doesn't seem to notice if any of us are home, as long as his food dish is full and his cat box is emptied regularly.

It used to be that all my children wanted was *Mama, Mama, Only Mama*, and they were permanently affixed to my hip. Now, they'll choose to stay home with SigO as opposed to running errands with me. (Unless, of course, they get to buy something.) But the best thing I've done for their relationship with SigO is to go out of town.

Even though we've lived together for several years, I was resistant to leaving the kids alone with him overnight. He felt that I didn't trust him, but that wasn't it—it was yet another reaction to my own childhood. I only saw my father on summer vacations, and he'd often go out of town with my brother and leave me in the care of whatever stepmother I had at the time, and I hated it. I only get the kids four nights a week, so I try my hardest never to schedule events or workshops when I have them, unless I can bring them along. I've dragged my kids to a few literary events and conferences, and while it would certainly be easier to leave them at home, I was loath to do so. But after the release of my first memoir I had to do some promotional events when I had the kids, and now that they're older, missing school is a much bigger deal than it used to be, so I recently left them home with SigO while I went on a twenty-hour trip to Boston.

SigO took them for fast food. He found Aesop's Fables to read them at bedtime. He got Big Pants to school on time and encouraged Tiny Pants to ride his bike alone to school for the very first time, which he absolutely loved. When I got home, the boys were happy to see me, but they didn't wrap themselves around my legs and beg me never to leave again.

That night at bedtime, Tiny Pants wouldn't go to bed until SigO came upstairs, too.

"I can't sleep unless you hit me with the baseball bat!" Tiny Pants said.

"Don't say that," Big Pants reprimanded.

"But I like to be hit with the baseball bat," Tiny Pants said, as SigO took the Nerf bat and gently pounded his back with it.

"But you're overly dramatic, and I don't want you to write a book someday and say that SigO hit you with a baseball bat every night," Big Pants said. And that's when I knew we weren't a Venn diagram, but a family.

Fourth of July as a Single Parent

The orange life-flight helicopter kicked off the Mayville parade, flying low over the parade route. It was followed by vintage fire trucks, marching bands, Cub Scouts, and all the expected Fourth of July participants. After the parade, we walked to the park where there was live music, kids' activities, and a line to see inside the helicopter. I balanced the baby on my hip as my three-year-old son looked very carefully at everything. A nurse in an orange flight suit explained the equipment, including a box of Nilla Wafers for "cookie emergencies." She asked my son if he wanted a cookie, but he wordlessly shook his head.

"Why didn't you want a cookie?" I asked. I don't think I had ever seen him refuse a cookie before.

"They are for emergencies. I wasn't having an emergency," he replied.

That was the last Fourth of July I spent with my boys.

We were supposed to alternate holidays every year, but I had a strategy of being agreeable. When my ex asked to have them two years in a row, I said yes, because I knew I would want a favor one day. I figured being easygoing would create a stockpile of goodwill I could draw on later, but then it became a tradition. Every year my ex took our boys back to his home town of Chicago for the Fourth of July. I understood. He came from a large and fun family that had a massive party every year. They even made their own family parade and walked around the neighborhood. I wanted my kids to have an abundance of cousins and aunts and uncles.

But I missed them.

Terribly.

When I was a child, Fourth of July was right up there with Christmas and Halloween—way above Easter and Thanksgiving. It was everything good and Norman Rockwell–esque about America. The parade was two blocks from our house. The all-day festival and fireworks an easy bike ride away. Our Fourth of July parties were only a handful of people, but they were people that were dear to me.

Every year that my kids were gone I pretended that it would be OK, and every year it wasn't. Finally, I wrote off what was probably an overly harsh email to Daddy Pants demanding that he allow me to take the kids the following year on the Fourth of July. I knew I couldn't compete with his family, but I wanted to take my kids to a parade and buy red helium balloons from a hawker and tie the string around a little tanned wrist, just like my mother did for me. My ex-husband, perhaps following his own strategic plan of agreeability, agreed without argument.

Except then I got accepted into an MFA program, and their residencies were over the Fourth of July holiday. I had to write Daddy Pants back and ask if he would ignore my not-so-friendly email and instead arrange his schedule to take the kids for the next two Fourth of Julys, and also the next two New Year's Eves. He readily agreed, and for the next two years, he scheduled his vacations around my schooling. After that, I couldn't interfere with what had become my children's Fourth of July tradition.

I understood the importance of traditions to children. I knew that the one year I broke with my tradition of spending Christmas at my mother's and instead went to my father's house, it was the bleakest holiday of my childhood. It wasn't that he did anything wrong, mind you, but it wasn't *the same*. So I am aware that

(continued)

removing my kids from their annual Chicago celebration will likely end in disappointment for everyone. I don't want to be the one who ruined their holiday with my insistence of togetherness.

One year I got lucky, and my neighborhood had a parade on the Saturday preceding the Fourth of July. We didn't just march in the parade waving flags—we made a 4 x 4 float complete with four-foot-tall sit-on ponies and I pulled the children down the street while they held flags. One wore his baseball uniform, and the other dressed inexplicably as a Canadian Mountie. They felt too shy to wave their flags, and I didn't make them. Afterward we ate cookies and accepted our "best float" award. (We were the only float.) We planned to do this every year, but the neighborhood moved their parade to the actual Fourth of July in the following years, and the boys were always gone for it.

Once again this year I will do grown-up things on the Fourth of July. There are some benefits to being child-free on the holiday. You don't have to remain sober and can tell as many ribald jokes as you like. You don't have to quite so vigilant if drunk people set off fireworks. I will bake a dessert, go to a party, drink festive drinks, and probably even wear red, white, and blue. I may even go down to the fireworks and sit among other people's families, but my heart will still be in Chicago, where my boys are.

Tomorrow I will once again enjoy the peace and quiet that comes from having my boys on vacation with their father. I'll get work done and not be interrupted with the constant summer refrains of "I'm bored!" or "My brother's making me crazy!" There are benefits to the kids being out of town, as well. But today, I will miss those little creatures and fake a smile for my neighbors. If I hold the smile long enough, it might start to feel like I mean it.

Posted by Lara Lillibridge July 4, 2017 at 10:32 AM
More: U.S. News, Arts and Entertainment, Toddlers, Chicago, Walking, Mayville

Grade A

SigO and I were watching Netflix around ten o'clock one night when I got a text from a mother of one of Big Pants's friends.

"I saw your ex the other day. Wow."

Hmm. I was unsure what that meant. Luckily, she clarified.

"He's a hottie—Grade A."

Um, OK? Really? How was I supposed to react to that? Offer to hook her up—wait, she's married. Does this mean she thinks I have good taste? Or that I was stupid to divorce him? And she's met my SigO and made no comment, so does that mean she's being respectful of my current relationship, or that she thinks I downgraded?

Here's the weird thing—people don't usually react to my ex like that. Like me, he's not exactly a head-turner, though he grows on you. I'm not disparaging him—he has naturally straight teeth that never needed braces, 20/20 vision with nice blue eyes, ears that don't stick out (and detached earlobes, obviously) and a strong cleft chin. He's not very tall, nor was he unusually muscular. Daddy Pants is solid, reasonably attractive, and when we got along I found him quite cute, but I don't think anyone has ever whistled as he walked by, though I guess women don't wolf-whistle men all that often anyway. He also didn't go in for flashy douchebaggery fashion—no hair gel (not that he had enough hair to gel) or trendy clothes. He wore Dockers and polos, Levi's jeans and ironed T-shirts—solid, like I said.

SigO, on the other hand, has a distinctive look. His hair is nearly down to his elbows, and whether you care for that look or not—I have loved long-haired weirdos since high school—you notice him. He gets plenty of attention when we go out together—sometimes from men, admittedly, who assume from behind that he is a woman—but plenty of random drunk women have braided his hair at bars. I am used to that. Daddy Pants, though, well, my friend's reaction was a first. It was late when she texted, though, so I chalked it up to wine-o-clock and tried to forget it.

A few months later, she brought it up again. "I know, awkward that I think your ex is a hottie . . ." she texted. Um, ya think? This time, it was during the workday, and I knew she was sober. Well, I guess I didn't really know for sure that she was sober, but she didn't seem like a day drinker. I remained unsure how to respond, and whether or not I should tell Daddy Pants. Maybe he'd be flattered. Maybe he'd feel weird when he ran into her at school functions. I bided my time and bit my tongue. Keeping my mouth shut doesn't come naturally to me. Daddy Pants and I sat next to each other at baseball games. Should I tell him? No. Not yet. Save it. Hold the story back. You never know when you may need it. I'm not exactly sure why I might need a story about a mother calling him Grade A, but it could happen. My motivation could even be pure—say, he needed an ego boost or distraction from something I'd done that irritated him, like when I drive over his lawn at drop-off.

Circling Hope

Tiny Pants is a collector, and he loves to work on his collection at any opportunity—perusing catalogs and looking online for things to add to his stash, and then artfully displaying them all over the floor and in piles by his bed. In his opinion, the house exists as a museum for his collection, and since we still have room left on the floor, there's no reason to stop adding to it. What does he collect, you ask? New things. Sticks. Rocks. Stuffed animals. Things That Might Come in Handy Someday.

We've tried to squelch this shopping obsession, but unfortunately, both Daddy Pants and I are shoppers at heart, and he has our DNA, so it's a hard-fought battle. Let's be honest—buying stuff is fun. The problem is that Tiny doesn't have a job capable of providing the resources he needs to support his acquisition habit.

But I got a ray of hope this year. When the Christmas catalogs started arriving, he went through and circled everything he wanted, but for the first time, he circled gifts he wanted to give to others as well as things he wanted gifted to him. A curio shelf shaped like the whale from *Hitchhiker's Guide to the Galaxy* for my brother, a mercury ball for SigO, and something unknown and magical (I'm sure) for me, though I promised not to look. Of course, it will be hard to buy him anything in the catalog if everyone who has access to credit cards can't see what he circled, but that's a technicality.

I knew I was finally growing up when I was more excited about people opening the gifts I gave them than I was about opening gifts I received. I think it took me until I was in junior high before Christmas became about giving more than receiving. At nine, Tiny is ahead of the game. Sure, he mostly circled things for himself, but who doesn't?

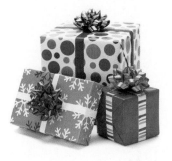

When Nana and Grandma Pat came for Christmas this year, he raced to the tree. I started to reprimand him to slow down, not to just grab a present for himself, but I held off for a moment, not wanting to ruin Christmas. Christmas was for the children first and foremost. I figured the first thing he'd grab the would be the biggest present with his name on it—that's what I would have done at his age.

He knelt by the tree, bent nearly in half as he dug below the artificial pine branches. He pulled out the presents he bought for Nana and Grandma Pat and thrust the sparkly boxes at them. He sat back on his heels, grinning as widely as he did as a toothless baby. He ignored the present addressed to him I tried to place in his hands, leaning forward to help his grandmas unwrap the presents he bought them.

Tell-All: I Make a Turkey for No Good Reason (Includes a Bonus Cranberry Sauce Recipe)

While I had been fine microwaving food for the kids and myself for all of my single-mama years, SigO had this expectation for marginally edible food that everyone would eat, as referenced in the chicken casserole standoff. Being both lazy and unskilled, I discovered the joy of the pre-measured (but not precooked) box dinner. There are several places that deliver all the necessary ingredients to make a more than marginally edible meal along with step-by-step instructions with photos. It turns out almost every meat is cooked in olive oil with salt and pepper, topped with an interesting sauce—so although the basics are the same, somehow they are all slightly different. I have finally learned to zest, slurry, and mince. As this book winds down, I find my cooking is getting more grown-up—at least on occasion. With my pocket googler in one hand and wooden spoon in the other I've become somewhat domesticated. Today I voluntarily cooked a turkey breast for no occasion at all.

My grocery store has this pick-up option. I go online, select my items, and for the low price of $4.95 someone collects them, bags them, and loads them in the car for me. This is a life-changing miracle. The downside is that I'm not exactly good at paying attention to quantity. Once I accidentally wound up with eleven apples instead of four, another time I ended up with only ¼ pound of beef for four people. This week, I somehow ordered an eight-pound turkey, which was about double the size I needed. In my defense, they may not actually sell smaller turkey breasts. Since I didn't go inside the store, I have no idea what size turkeys even come in.

Turkey

Ingredients

Turkey breast: the kind where someone has amputated the legs already

½ cup sugar

¾ cup salt

Spices of your choosing (more on this will be revealed later)

Butter (I used half a stick, which was too much, but after smearing a stick of butter on a raw turkey it didn't seem reusable.)

Time. Not thyme. I mean, you need to plan this one out a few hours/days in advance. I had no thyme, as you will read shortly.

Procedure

The night before I lovingly placed my turkey carcass into a bath of 9 cups of water with ¾ cup of salt and ½ cup sugar and tucked it into the fridge to spend the night (12–24 hours). I didn't have a big enough bowl, so I used my largest pot.

Now that I was ready to cook the turkey, I first had to decide on a pan. I somehow or other acquired an official two-part roasting pan that had a tray-topper thing with a zillon holes in the top that sat on top of a bottom pan/dripping catcher. Unfortunately, the one time I had used it previously, it was a bitch to clean. At this point, you are familiar with how much I hate cleaning, so I covered my roasting pan tray-topper thing with tinfoil, then poked holes in it using a pen while the oven preheated. I had hoped that this way, the juices could drain and it would be easier to clean. Don't do this. The tinfoil stuck to the top part of the roaster pan, and then I had to peel off strips of greasy tinfoil with my fingers. File this under "It seemed like a good idea at the time."

According to two sources on the internet, one should preheat the oven to 450, then reduce the heat to either 325 or 250 (depending on who you ask) the minute you put the bird in the oven. No real explanation was given for this baffling phenomenon. My turkey's packaging instructed me to cook it at 325, so I preheated at 450 and turned it down to 325 when I put the turkey in the oven.

Next, I did something I swear I would never do. *I actually went under the skin.* I have never been willing to touch a carcass more than absolutely necessary, but I wanted to take my cooking skills to the next level. I had to snip away the weird stretchy connecting membrane from the carcass at the bottom in one place, but then I was able to forcibly run my fingers under the skin, while saying over and over, "Don't think of it as skin, think of it as an interesting substance. Don't think of it as skin, think of it as an interesting substance." Once it was loosened, I was all set.

Next, I over-melted a stick of butter in the microwave. I thought I had read somewhere that 19 seconds would soften butter without melting it, but it turns out that 15 seconds was a little too long. So instead of rubbing the turkey with softened butter, I sort of spilled melted butter on top of the skin and rubbed it around with my fingers. It turns out that when hot butter meets cold turkey skin, it immediately coagulates into solid butter again, which was handy. Next, I pulled up the skin and shoved some butter underneath, but only a little because the whole touching the skin thing was starting to be a little more than I could handle.

I washed my hands two or three times because butter + raw turkey = eww. Next, I went to my spice cabinet while singing, "parsley, sage, rosemary, and thyme," which I pronounced as th-ime because that was how I sang it as a little girl and it is my house and no one else was in the room to

(continued)

correct me. However, I had neither parsley nor sage. Only rosemary. I did have crystalized lime, garlic, and cilantro seasoning, and since it wasn't actually Thanksgiving, I didn't have to feel constrained by tradition—not that I feel constrained by tradition very often in my life, anyway. The lime seasoning stuff said it was for rice, vegetables, fish, chicken, pork, and beef. It did not specifically say that it was for turkey, but I felt that was exclusionary bullshit and I wasn't going to buy into their prejudicial restrictions.

One culinary thing my mother taught me was to sniff spices and if they smell good together, they will taste good together, so I sniffed the garlic-lime stuff and the rosemary. They did not smell right together, so I ditched the rosemary.

Now, I have a theory about spices and turkey: no matter what spices you use or what you stuff it with, it always tastes pretty much the same. You can stuff it with oranges, like my first-ex-husband liked to do. You can carefully layer slices of apples on top of the breast like tiny turkey armor, as a houseguest did one year. No matter what spices you choose, it all winds up tasting like turkey. I sprinkled the breast with salt, pepper, and the lime-garlic stuff, and then I peeled back the skin once again and threw some spices up in there in a random/chaotic fashion because I was at my limit of skin touching. I adjusted the wire rack so it was at the bottom-third position in the oven, and slid the pan in. I actually remembered to knock the heat down to 325. Everyone—both my ex-husbands, the internet-at-large, and the plastic turkey wrapping—all agree that turkey needs to be cooked for twenty minutes a pound. They all also agree that one should check the turkey with a meat thermometer, but I don't own one, so I went with the cut-into-it-and-look method I am so fond of.

The downside of turkey is the prep before cooking. The upside of a turkey breast is that it needs no basting, so basically it was a shove-it-in-the-oven-and-ignore-it type of meal. (I do recommend looking at it periodically, and if the skin starts to brown too much, cover it with a tinfoil tent.) Since it wasn't actually Thanksgiving, I didn't feel any pressure to provide excessive side dishes. Bob Evans premade mashed potatoes, a jar of gravy, and some corn on the cob that had been rattling around my fridge for a week worked just fine. Oh, I did make cranberry sauce, because unlike jarred gravy, which is so good that there is no earthly reason to make it from scratch, homemade cranberry sauce is far superior to the stuff in a can, and only takes 10 minutes.

Cranberry Sauce

Ingredients
1 bag of fresh cranberries (They come in a standard size.)
1 cup orange juice
1 cup sugar

Procedure
Heat juice and sugar in pot on stove, stirring until dissolved. Add cranberries and stir occasionally. When cranberries pop open (roughly 5–10 minutes), remove from heat. Sauce will thicken upon cooling. I wasn't sure what they meant by this whole cooling thing, so I shoved it in the fridge until dinnertime. Note: you really need to wait for all the cranberries to pop, not just some of them. However, if you removed it from heat before they all popped, you will have less firm cranberry sauce, but you get to pop them with your teeth, and that is incredibly satisfying.

Wait, Don't Ride Off So Quickly!

I turned around, and Big Pants became a tween. It's my fault, I guess. He's had a cell phone—old school flip-style, where you have to use a number pad to text—for several years, since his first overnight school trip. I couldn't bear to send him without some sort of lifeline. (For me, of course. I knew he'd be fine.) And although he's had this phone since fourth grade, he's never cared much about it, until he changed schools. Now he suddenly has friends who text, and I upgraded him to a smartphone to make group texts more manageable. Suddenly I only saw the top of my son's head as his eyes became glued to his pocket friend communication device. Now, it's a nice enough head and all, I'm rather fond of it, but I like his eyes and those endearing freckles across the bridge of his nose a little bit more. The top of the head is not particularly good at expressions and looks basically the same every day.

In addition to introducing the pocket texting device, I bought him a bike so that he can go visit his friends without me, because I am inherently a very lazy person. Except that whole "go places without your mother" idea is way more appealing to him than I anticipated. He's all in for ditching me and his little brother, which I support in theory, but not so much in practice.

I miss him. He's quickly riding off into the world without me—which is as it should be at his age—but I didn't think I'd feel lonely being left behind.

Oh sure, it's fine for his little brother to miss him, but mothers are supposed to be tough. We want our children to take the next step toward independence, except some of us don't really entirely want them to leave us behind. I was unprepared for this, even though I instigated it.

He skipped a grade in school last year, and he's jumped up in maturity to match it. His tooth fell out, and he didn't mention the tooth fairy. The molar is still sitting abandoned in the kitchen several months later. (Hoarding old teeth is really kind of weird and creepy if you think about it, but I'm not sure exactly what to do with the ziplock bag containing a tooth. Seems callous to throw it away.) He went on a sleepover and didn't bring his pillow pet or teddy bear. He suddenly has an opinion on clothing: "I won't wear shorts without pockets, Mama." As soon as school was out for the summer, some sort of maturity switch was flipped and he automatically started acting like the high school freshman he's about to become. I'm not sure what happened between May 30 and June 6, but it feels like he grew up an entire year in the course of a week, and I love it and hate it all at the same time.

I watch him as he sits on his ten-speed, pushes off with one foot, coasts down the driveway, and turns right. I remember when he insisted he didn't need to learn how to ride a bike and was just going to ride his scooter for the rest of his life. I remember the first time he rode without training wheels, how he crashed in a ditch and got a bruise the size of his fist in the middle of his chest. I remember all the failed family bike rides when one kid crashed into the other, and they fought about who had to ride in front, and we made it three blocks before someone was bleeding and someone else was crying and I just gave up and we all came home and didn't try it again for another year.

I watch him pedal and remember all the days upon days when he was three and four and five, when I wondered if I would live through the toddler years of playing trains and ani-
mals and mess a foot deep in the living room, action figures with legs chewed off by the dog, a sink always overflow-ing with dirty dishes, and boys who wanted nothing to do with sleeping ever. I remember letting him sit on my

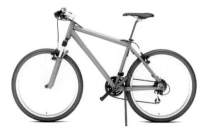

lap to do his homework every night, because I wanted him to love school and think it was important, and how his little fingers felt wrapped around my back as he slept at night in my bed—his own bed empty and ignored.

I am proud, too, of the boy he's become. He never hits his brother or complains about homework. He doesn't talk back and I love to watch him play baseball, gloved hand at the ready as he protects third base, calling "two outs, plays at first," to his teammates, his "r" soft and slightly Bostonian sounding, echoing the child who couldn't form his consonants properly. I've watched him stand in his suit in front of a real judge and argue and win his mock trial case, and clapped as he walked across the stage to receive academic awards.

I watch him ride until he reaches the bend in the road and turns out of sight. There's nothing left to do but go back inside. Everyone says children grow up fast. I just never thought it would be quite this quickly.

MODERN PARENTS MESSY KIDS

Should You Send Your Ex a Father's Day Card?

This will be our tenth Father's Day since the divorce, and just like every other year, I'll take my two sons to the store and help them pick out gifts for their father.

Some years I'm surprised I didn't get lockjaw from forcing myself to smile as I helped them wrap their presents, and I can't say I've never stooped to passive-aggressive gifting. (Please don't ask me about the garden gnome.)

It wasn't always a joy to spend money on my ex-husband, particularly since I was mothering on a tight budget for a lot of years. But it was important to me. I wanted my boys to learn to be thoughtful, generous, and that it's important to make the effort to show someone you love that they matter.

Every year I've provided paper and markers and cold, hard cash, and I've patiently helped my kids make good buying decisions. I've handed them tape and held the scissors while they wrapped their presents. But there was always something about Father's Day that nagged at me.

Kids aren't the only people to give fathers cards. Wives give them to their husbands, too.

In perusing Father's Day cards, I found several themes that I could relate to:

(continued)

1. **Whoa—look at what a great job we're doing. Our kids are awesome.**
   Our kids are amazing, well-adjusted creatures. They are outstanding and resilient humans and, so far, seem to be emerging mostly unscathed from the divorce. That's worth celebrating.

2. **I appreciate the father-things you do (at least most of the time).**
   My ex-husband is not the right man for me, but he is the right father for our children. He's never stood them up or begged off visitation time—he's always been someone solid they can count on. He changed diapers, went to excruciatingly long school concerts, and dealt with puking children on his own, just like I did.

3. **Thanks for making my life easier!**
   My ex has also used vacation days to watch the kids so I could go out of town for work conferences. We call and text each other to discuss the children multiple times a week. We still co-parent together, even if we haven't lived together in nearly a decade.

4. **You are the man and we'd be so screwed without you.**
   OK, the whole "you're the man" thing is *not* something I can get behind, but if he were to die or move away, the kids would be devastated. If the kids are devastated, you can pretty much bet my misery will increase as well.

5. **We've come a long way, baby!**
   Even in the first year when we could barely be civil to each other, he texted, *"If you are ever on the ledge, you can call me. I may hate you, but the kids need a mother as well as a father."* This year I got my first Mother's Day text from him: *"Happy Mother's Day. You are a good mom to them."* We've come a long way as a non-couple. We both single-parented two kids in diapers half the week, when neither kid would sleep alone

in their beds. We've done first days of kindergarten together as divorced parents and this fall we'll be doing first day of high school pictures with our eldest.

We don't always agree on what's best for the kids, and we don't really have a friendship consisting of friendly banter or easy small talk. But we've both tried to put these two boys first in our lives and kept our own issues out of our children's sight. And I may be wrong, but I feel that's Father's Day card-worthy.

Of course, I can't really send him a card. He'd think it would be awkward and weird and he'd be right. But this year, I think I'll send him a heartfelt text that says it all: Happy Father's Day. And I'll mean it.

. . . .

Posted by Lara Lillibridge May 29, 2018

Saying Farewell to Only Mama

It's been four years since I have been a single mama. The Pants brothers now have three active parental units, making them parentally privileged or burdened, depending on the day and who you ask. As much as I love writing about my boys, I wouldn't have wanted to have a mommy blogger for a parent during my high school years. I think it is time to draw this book to a close, and give the kids some much deserved privacy. Besides, I wrote much more freely before they learned how to read. This fall, I have agonized over the ethics of writing about my kids as they became more and more adult-like, and I've decided that there will be no discourse on their first pimples or first dates. They have the right to experience life without worrying about it being preserved for all time on the internet. It is time for me to find a new source of material. So farewell, kind readers, and thanks for all the support and encouragement you have given us all these years.

—*Only Mama*

Acknowledgments

Thanks to my children for giving me their blessing to write about them—and also for providing me with so much material. Thanks to my parents for all their support during those early years. Huge thanks to Chamois Holschuh at Skyhorse Publishing for believing in my beloved and somewhat zany little book and to my beta reader crew, in chronological order: Sandy Roffey, Sherry Dove, Maria Sabala, Kathleen Lenane, and Elizabeth Collins. I'll always be grateful to my Debutante Ball cohorts as well: Julie Clark, Kimmery Martin, Cass Morris, Kaitlyn Patterson, and the previous classes of Debs—you helped get me through both my debut and sophomore memoirs. And of course, to SigO, always.

Author's Note

"Step Stools" previously appeared in *Vandalia: The Arts Journal of West Virginia Wesleyan College*, vol. 14: 2014.

The following posts first appeared on *Good Men Project*:
- "What a Boy's Love of Baseball Taught His Sports-Averse Mother"
- "What If We Treated Marriage More Like the Contract It Is?"

The following posts first appeared on *Huffington Post*:
- "Sometimes You Are Not a Victim—Your Are an Asshole"
- "Elephant Skin, Grinning Corpse Face, and Fighting Gravity"
- "A Divorced Mom Talks to Her Children about Marriage"
- "Fourth of July as a Single Parent"
- "Saying Farewell to the Tooth Fairy"

A shortened version of "How I Became a Hockey Mom Against My Better Judgment" appeared on *Modern Parents, Messy Kids*.

"Should You Send Your Ex a Father's Day Card?" first appeared on *Modern Parents, Messy Kids*.